Occupational Thera   nd
Life Course Deve'   nt

This book is dedicated to our families, who continue to make our journeys through the life course both pleasurable and fascinating:

David Sugarman, Clare Sugarman
Erica Sugarman and George Faulkner

Mike Wright, Kate Wright
Hannah and Peter Lamb
George Wright and Ellie Bradshaw

We would also like to dedicate this book to the memory of our mothers, who taught us so much about managing the life course, with all its ups and downs, twists and turns:

Leonie Helene Heppenstall

Margaret Halsey

Occupational Therapy and Life Course Development:

A Work Book for Professional Practice

Ruth Wright and Léonie Sugarman

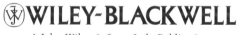
WILEY-BLACKWELL

A John Wiley & Sons, Ltd., Publication

Library of Congress Cataloging-in-Publication Data

Wright, Ruth.
Occupational therapy and life course development : a work book for professional practice / Ruth Wright and Léonie Sugarman.
p. ; cm.
Includes bibliographical references and index.
ISBN 978-0-470-02545-1 (pbk. : alk. paper) 1. Occupational therapy. 2. Life cycle, Human. I. Sugarman, Léonie, 1950-II. Title.
[DNLM: 1. Occupational Therapy. 2. Life Change Events. WB 555 W952o 2009]
RM735.W75 2009
615.8′515–dc22
2008044756

A catalogue record for this book is available from the British Library.

Set in 10.5 on 13 pt Palatino by SNP Best-set Typesetter Ltd., Hong Kong
Printed in Singapore by Markono Print Media Pte Ltd

1 2008

Contents

Contents

Preface

Although it contains plenty of text, *Occupational Therapy and Life Course Development* is not a textbook. It is, as its subtitle indicates, a work book for professional practice. You will need to work through the book fairly systematically if you are to get maximum benefit from it. This may sound like something of a chore, but we hope that you will find the process sufficiently interesting to make it engaging, and even exciting. *Occupational Therapy and Life Course Development* is designed to introduce life course concepts in an applied way, to help you to reflect on your learning and your individual experience, and to enable you to undertake your learning in a way that suits you.

We come from a combined academic and practice background, our subject and practice areas being in one case occupational therapy and in the other psychology. We also have backgrounds in counselling and family therapy, but both now work as academics and educators. We have chosen to write a book like this for a number of reasons. The first and most important reason is that we believe a working knowledge of life course theory can significantly enhance your practice in the health and social care arena by helping you to be more client-centred: seeing individuals holistically and in context in a way that will help your decision-making and your ability to focus on the issues that are important to those with whom you are working.

Health and social care practitioners, including occupational therapists, are now working much more generically and independently than ever before, and increasingly as lone workers outside the NHS, social services or other traditional employers. The *Choosing Health* agenda (Department of Health, 2004) and the imperatives arising from equality and diversity legislation are key drivers in all health and social care workplaces. Similarly, across all health and social care professions, evidence of continuing professional development is a requirement for remaining registered. *Occupational Therapy and Life Course Development* attempts to address a range of relevant professional concerns. Specifically:

- The book provides a tool to help both students and qualified practitioners develop and enhance a framework for their practice that supports all individuals and settings in a holistic and inclusive way.
- The interactive nature of the book promotes lifelong learning for continuing professional development. Independent learning that can be accessed flexibly by individuals or groups is the mode of delivery. This taps into current demands made by both education and practice. Using this book could be taken as evidence of continuing professional development, a requirement for all health and social care practitioners wishing to remain registered with the College of Occupational Therapists or similar registering body.
- Our emphasis is on the individual needs of clients within their own specific context. This marks a move away from an emphasis on traditional delivery settings, and supports both the equality and diversity agenda and the need to address public health issues in terms of individual health needs and choices.

You will find that much of this book is organized as a work book based on a single case study. It includes theory related to lifespan development and managing change, and exercises for readers to complete in order to apply the theory to their practice (albeit hypothetical practice when it is the case study that is the focus of attention).

Writing this book has kept us occupied for some considerable time, and, like the life course itself, it has been a journey of discovery and adventure. It has been a long, and not always easy, journey, and one replete with lows as well as highs, setbacks as well as advances. Nonetheless, we got there in the end! We very much hope that your journey through this book will be both rewarding and enjoyable – at least most of the time.

Léonie Sugarman and Ruth Wright
September 2008

0. *Read Me: It All Starts Here*

We have called this element of the book Chapter 0 rather than 'Introduction' because, as advised by Doyle (2003), we want to do all that we can to ensure you do not skip it. We are both educators, and are well aware of the temptation to ignore the aperitif in order to get to the main course of the text. This chapter, however, is more than an hors d'oeuvre that can be taken or left depending on your level of interest or commitment. Without this vital first chapter, you will not be able to take full advantage of the interactive element of this book.

The book is designed as an interactive text. Through a series of Learning Tasks, it is hoped that you will be encouraged to reflect actively and think critically about your role and work as a health and social care professional. Some of the tasks invite you to reflect on concepts and issues in relation to your own personal or professional life. Other tasks ask you to analyse points in relation to one or more people in the case study that is outlined later in this chapter (p. 6). Through this case study, we have striven to ground theoretical and abstract concepts in a concrete and practical example that reflects at least some of the complexities that make up the fabric of clients' lives. We suggest that you set aside an A4-sized notebook or spring-bound file specifically as a Learning Journal to accompany this text. In it, you should record both your responses to the Learning Tasks that permeate the book and any notes you make on the topics under discussion. The intention is that it will provide you with a useful and interesting record of your thoughts and how they developed during the course of working through this book.

The experiential learning cycle and personal learning styles

Taken together, the text of this book, the structured questions and activities, and your own experience in your training and practice, should propel you round all four stages of the experiential learning cycle (Kolb *et al.*, 2001; Kolb & Kolb, 2005). This model sees learning as a continuous, four-stage cyclical process, as shown in Figure 0.1, in which immediate *concrete experience* provides the basis for *reflection and observation*. Theories, hypotheses or *abstract concepts* are developed from these observations, and these concepts are then tested through *active experimentation*. The testing gives rise to a new *concrete experience*, and the cycle begins to repeat itself. In fact, since the new experience is different from that which initiated the learning cycle in the first place, the model would be better represented as a spiral rather than a circle.

Through reading the text of this book and completing its Learning Tasks, we hope that you will engage with all four of Kolb's (1984) different learning modes: active, reflective, abstract and concrete. We believe it is this that will enable you to develop an active understanding of life course issues, which you will be able to draw on creatively to enhance your practice. Each phase of the learning cycle places different demands on you, such that you must alternate between affective and conceptual experiencing, and between reflective and active involvement. These alternate emphases are repre-

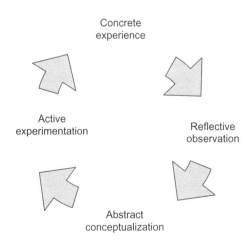

Concrete
experience

Active
experimentation

Reflective
observation

Abstract
conceptualization

Fig. 0.1 The experiential learning cycle (Kolb, 1984; Kolb and Kolb, 2005)

sented in the vertical and horizontal dimensions of Figure 0.1. We know that, whilst, ideally, we would cycle through all of these learning modes, in reality we often tend to have distinct preferences for a particular way – or style – of learning that emphasizes some phases of the learning cycle at the expense of others. Explore this point further by completing Learning Task 0.1. It provides a framework for thinking about your own learning style preferences and strengths, and the styles you might have overlooked or failed to develop.

Learning Task 0.1   My preferred ways of learning

There are four groups of questions below, with each group relating to a different 'learning mode', or stage in the learning process. For each item, score:

• 2 points if it is highly characteristic of you
• 1 point if it is somewhat characteristic of you
• 0 points if it is not at all characteristic of you.

Concrete Experience: feeling

1. ___ I rely on feelings when making decisions
2. ___ I act on hunches and 'gut reactions'
3. ___ I learn from personal experience
4. ___ I have strong feelings
5. ___ I tend to be open about how I'm feeling
6. ___ I seek personal meaning in what I learn
7. ___ I learn through interacting with others
8. ___ I like to face up to my emotions
9. ___ I like to focus on immediate, here-and-now experiences
10. ___ I am an emotional person

TOTAL FOR *CE* ___

Reflective Observation: watching

1. ___ I learn best by watching and reflecting
2. ___ I tend to think about possible outcomes before trying something new
3. ___ I listen carefully when wanting to learn something
4. ___ I am quiet and reflective
5. ___ I take my time before making decisions

6. ___ I like to consider all sides of an argument
7. ___ I seek out background information on issues
8. ___ I like to watch others before having a go myself
9. ___ I am careful to avoid jumping to conclusions
10. ___ I am an imaginative person

TOTAL FOR *RO* ___

Abstract Conceptualization: thinking

1. ___ I tend to reason and think things through
2. ___ I like information to be presented in an organized, logical fashion
3. ___ I rely on logical thinking when making decisions
4. ___ I am an 'ideas person'
5. ___ I evaluate things
6. ___ I like ideas and theories
7. ___ I probe the logic behind ideas
8. ___ I seek a conceptual understanding of what I learn
9. ___ I formulate plans and hypotheses
10. ___ I am an analytic person

TOTAL FOR *AC* ___

Active Experimentation: doing

1. ___ I like to apply ideas to new situations
2. ___ I test ideas by trying them out
3. ___ I will often 'throw caution to the wind'
4. ___ I like to set my own goals
5. ___ I tend to talk rather than listen
6. ___ I work by trial-and-error and learn from my mistakes
7. ___ I adapt what I learn for my own uses
8. ___ I am good at implementing decisions
9. ___ I enjoy participating in something new
10. ___ I am an active person

TOTAL FOR *AE* ___

If you add up your scores for each learning mode, you will get an idea of your own learning mode preferences – the higher the score, the stronger the preference. You will also have an indication of which learning modes you least prefer.

Please note that this is not a systematically designed measure of preferred learning styles. For that you would need to complete a standardized inventory, such as Kolb's (1999) *Learning Styles Inventory* or Honey and Mumford's (2006) *Learning Styles Questionnaire*. The present activity is designed as a catalyst to encourage you to think about and develop your learning skills. Your own learning preferences and strengths will be a great asset to you as an occupational therapist or other type of health or social care professional – but guard against overusing your strengths. You will become a better-rounded practitioner if you can also develop your skills in your less preferred learning modes. We hope that this work book will help you in this process.

As a final activity before leaving this Learning Task, turn to your Learning Journal and jot down some reflections on completing this activity. What have you learnt about yourself from completing it? How might you develop and utilize your less preferred ways of learning? What could the benefit of this be?

You can do several things when armed with an insight into your own preferred learning style. First, you can seek out situations that enable you to give free rein to your preferences – in other words, situations that play to your strengths. Second, in recognition of the fact that all learning styles are important, you can seek out as co-workers those with a different learning style preference to yourself, that is aim for a balanced learning team. Third, and again in recognition that all learning styles and stages are important, you can seek to develop your own repertoire of learning skills by making a conscious effort to utilize and practise your currently underused and least developed styles. Whilst all of these strategies have their place, it is the third that we believe will be the most valuable in helping you to develop into a complete and well-rounded health and social care professional. Bear this in mind as you work through the different Learning Tasks in this work book.

Whilst a number of studies have been carried out that explore the preferred learning styles of occupational therapy students, their results have been somewhat contradictory and inconclusive. In one study (French *et al.*, 2007), the learning style preferences of occupational therapy students were spread across all four styles, with the most preferred style being one that involves the use of *concrete experience* and *reflective observation*. This contrasts with other studies, which have found a preference for *active experimentation* – in some instances combined with a preference for *concrete experience* (Kolb, 1984; Katz & Heimann, 1991; Linares, 1999) and in others with *abstract conceptualization* (Linares, 1999; Titiloye & Scott, 2001). Another study (Hauer *et al.*, 2005) found that occupational therapy students had a slight preference for *abstract conceptualization* and *reflective observation* in comparison to many other health care students. Again, however, preferences ranged across all learning styles. All of this suggests that occupational therapy attracts individuals with a range of learning style preferences, and this can be considered appropriate in a profession that offers a wide range of specialisms and ways of working. Furthermore, all practitioners in the health and social care field need to be able to learn from a variety of situations and experiences, and change their ways of working as new knowledge is discovered, reported and integrated into professional practice (French *et al.*, 2007). Strengthening and utilizing non-preferred learning styles is, therefore, a key professional skill.

The case study and its characters

Many of the Learning Tasks in this text relate to the case study that is summarized below. It is important that you become familiar with this case study now: you will need to refer back to it regularly in order to complete many of the guided activities in later chapters.

Case Study

Last month, while Andrew was away at university, his brother, Richard, found their mother, Helen, on the floor having suffered a right cardiovascular accident (CVA). Helen has now come home from hospital with mobility and fine-motor problems because of left-sided weakness. She is very tired and tearful. Helen is also having difficulty planning and ordering even familiar tasks. Her visual perception is confused. She does not want to talk about her situation.

Richard and Andrew recognized that their mother would need help and felt that her friends would be the best support. The family have lived in the area for 20 years and have a very strong local support network of neighbours, colleagues and friends they have met through shared activities, such as the school PTA, the horticultural club and a local book group. Mary, Helen's mother, however, wants only the family to be involved.

Case Study Characters

Helen Case is a 52-year-old woman who works as an infant school teacher. She lives in a four-bedroom 1970s house on an estate. It has a large garden, which Helen enjoys very much; she is a member of the local horticultural society. Helen and the family have good social networks on the estate. She also sings in the church choir and is a church visitor, which involves visiting older housebound church members to give them help and company on a regular basis. She is divorced and has two sons.

Andrew, Helen's elder son, is 21 years old and is in his last year at university in a major city some two hours' drive from home. On hearing of his mother's collapse, he responded by feeling sick, cold and disbelieving. He almost felt as though he were behaving heartlessly and feeling nothing; this has made him feel ashamed and guilty. He has been offered the opportunity to spend two years in the USA after graduation, undertaking further study and gaining work experience. He is now feeling much more upset about his mother's CVA. He no longer feels so stunned and is now wondering whether his planned visit to the USA will still be possible. He wants to go but does not want to leave his family unsupported. He finds this confusing and is inclined to feel angry.

Richard, Helen's younger son, is 18 years old and studying for A levels. He hopes to do an art foundation course locally next year. On finding his mother collapsed, Richard was horrified and in the following hours and days began to plan to leave school in order to look after her He put all his other plans on hold, gathered the family together and took on much of the care that Mary, his grandmother, needed. Richard is now beginning to seek more thought-through strategies for dealing with the situation, realizing that more balanced and longer-term strategies, which allow him some time away from the situation and leave plans for his own life open to him, are needed. He receives a lot of support from Andrew but is getting increasingly tired and low in mood.

John, Helen's ex-husband, has remarried but has no further children. John has contact with Andrew and Richard but is not generous to Helen with regard to financial contributions for them.

Mary, Helen's mother, is an active 77-year-old who also lives with them. Mary has been losing her sight over the last decade and now has very little vision indeed. She came to live with Helen after Helen's divorce, 12 years ago. Mary's husband, Helen's father, left the family when Helen was 13 and has had almost no contact with them thereafter, although he and Mary never actually divorced. He is still alive, but they have no contact details for him. Mary is terribly upset by Helen's CVA, having never considered that such a thing happened to people of Helen's age, let alone to her child. She fears that her impaired vision has put a strain on Helen that has affected her health. Mary is determined that the family will care for Helen as Helen has cared for them. She becomes angry at suggestions of outside help, and even wishes to refuse offers of assistance (for example with transport or shopping) from friends and neighbours. She writes to family members living far away, detailing the situation as she sees it and asking for support. She tries to persuade members of the family to promise a level of support that they cannot really offer, and frequently feels very frustrated and tearful. However, Mary is beginning to calm down a little as Helen is making a better physical recovery than she expected, and she believes that helping Helen to cope with her emotional state is something she is much more able to do.

The household also includes an elderly Jack Russell dog called **Wicket**.

Mary has two other children besides Helen:

Brian, the eldest, is 55 years old and married to **Elizabeth**; they have two children, a girl, **Laura**, aged 24, and a boy, **Mark**, aged 20. Brian is the very busy finance director of a large company and works abroad a lot. They are on good terms with Helen and her family, but contact is not frequent as Brian has little time to spare outside his job for anyone other than his immediate family. Elizabeth has put her energy into her own children, her own side of the family and life in her village. They live 250 miles away from Helen and Mary. Now that her children are growing up, Elizabeth accompanies Brian on trips abroad whenever possible. On hearing of Helen's CVA, both are very concerned, and Brian in particular is keen to help his mother and sister. He spends considerable time and energy investigating Helen's likely prognosis, contacting statutory, charitable and private services to see what may be available as help, and determines to visit more frequently. He wonders whether he should take charge of Mary's and Helen's financial arrangements. He does, however, after the initial shock, take the view that, whilst he must now maintain more contact with and take increased responsibility for his mother, nothing should be done in a hurry and it is Helen's wishes that matter the most. He also realizes that things may change over time.

Alison, Mary's youngest child, is 43 years old. Alison was a difficult teenager and was known to the local police from her mid-teens. She became pregnant aged 15, but the baby, a boy, **David**, was born prematurely and died at three days old. She married at 18 and had two daughters, Sarah and Katie, who are now 24 years old and 23 years old. She is divorced from her first husband and is now married to Paul; they have a son, Chris, aged nine. Alison works part-time at the local 7/11 shop.

Paul has no qualifications and gets casual work – usually labouring – when it is available. He tends to fall out with employers and very rarely holds a job for long. He drinks heavily and gets into fights and is well known to the police. He is, however, committed to Alison and the children and grandchildren, and Alison values this very much. She and Paul enjoy each other's company and have fun together going out to pubs and clubs, which is important to them. They live locally to Helen, although in another part of town, and move in a different community. They both, and Paul in particular, are very much a part of their own community, which includes Paul's extended family.

Sarah is a trained nurse; she works in the local hospital and is ambitious in her chosen career. She is close to her aunt Helen, but finds the contrast between Helen's life and Alison's difficult to come to terms with. She is married to a pharmacist, **Ranjiv**, and they have recently bought their own house in a village outside the town. Ranjiv is a British Asian whose family live in a town about 50 miles away. Although a traditional Hindu family, they accept Ranjiv's lifestyle and his marriage to Sarah, whom they like. Sarah has just discovered that she is pregnant. The pregnancy was not planned and Sarah is concerned about whether she will be able to cope with the competing demands of her career and motherhood. Sarah feels ambivalent about her parents and Katie. She loves them, but feels that they could do a lot better for themselves and that they should be more ambitious, especially for Chris, of whom she is very fond. She feels that they make excuses not to improve their lot and are rather disorganized.

She is somewhat ashamed of herself for feeling like this but also feels irritated with them. Nevertheless, she visits regularly and her family also visit her. However, Sarah feels closest to and most comfortable with her aunt, Helen. She has no contact with her father.

Katie lives with **Simon**. She works three nights a week at a local nursing home as a care assistant. Simon works as a scaffolder for a local firm; he is a steady worker and has been employed in the same firm for seven years. His family live locally and he has known Katie since she was 13 years old. She and Simon have two children, **Ben** and **Dan**, aged five and three years. Ben has just started attending the school where Chris is already a pupil and Dan goes to the local nursery five mornings a week. Katie and Simon plan to have more children: they would like a large family. They live in the same street as Alison and Paul and see a great deal of them and Paul's family. Alison and Paul help with childcare and babysitting. Katie and Simon are also close to Simon's family. Overall, they are a settled and contented couple, although Katie would like to get on better with Sarah and regrets the fact that she, like her sister, has no contact with her own father and that they have never really known him. Katie finds Sarah irritating and snobbish, and feels that Sarah slightly despises her. On learning of Helen's illness, Katie is determined to show her ability to help, and immediately begins to visit Helen daily or more, undertake cooking for Mary and Richard, and Andrew when he comes home from university (which he does immediately). Katie starts to formulate plans for undertaking almost all of her aunt's care, imagining that Helen will be able to do almost nothing for herself. She contacts social services to discover whether a house suitable for her own family and Helen's could be made available. Katie is already exhausted and beginning to feel that she is the only person taking her aunt's situation seriously.

Chris is at the local school, where he performs reasonably well academically, although he could probably do better. He is very good at football and running. He is a happy, popular boy, although he is sometimes in trouble as he finds concentrating difficult and can be a bit too lively in class. Paul, Sarah and Katie also attended this school. Chris is relaxed and accepting of all his family members. He goes to his grandmother's (Helen's) house one evening a week while Alison is working. He particularly enjoys playing with Wicket, the dog, on these evenings. He spends a lot of time with Paul's parents as they live near by, and Chris regards their house much as a second home. When he learns of Helen's illness, his first response is to go to Paul's parents and spend as much time as possible there. He does not want to talk about Helen but makes a lot of 'get well' cards for her. As time goes on, he is persuaded to visit her. He finds this difficult but has settled down to seeing her about once a week.

Family tree

Family trees, or genograms, are useful ways of representing a family (McGoldrick *et al.*, 1999), and your first activity is to construct a family tree for the Case family. Often presenting the family in a diagrammatic way gives insight into family dynamics and patterns, which may be clearer when presented in a visual form rather than as a narrative. Using symbols makes patterns easier to identify. Look now at Learning Task 0.2, and construct a genogram for the Case family.

Learning Task 0.2   A genogram of the Case family

Using the information in the case study, draw up a family tree for the full Case family. You can do this either on your own or together with a partner.

- You will need a:
  - pencil (much better than a pen as you will be able to rub out any mistakes)
  - rubber (see above)
  - blank page in your Learning Journal. Use the paper sideways (that is, landscape layout)
  - copy of the case study.

- Use the symbols below to indicate the relationships between the different family members:
  - ♀ female
  - ♂ male
  - ♀ or ♂ deceased
  - = married
  - – living with (as partner)
  - ‡ divorced or separated
  - | child of
  - ┊ adopted child of.

11

> When your genogram is complete, add the current ages (where known) of all the people included.
>
> Before returning to the text of the work book, take time to look closely at your genogram and note down any general or specific observations that occur to you. Try to identify any patterns that occur in the family.

Armed with your genogram and your initial impressions, you are now ready to begin thinking in earnest about life course theory and how it may help you in your professional practice as a health and social care professional.

1. *The Life Course as an Organizing Framework*

Whoever your clients are, one thing we can be sure of is that they will be somewhere on the path from cradle to grave, and that where they are in this journey is going to affect their needs. To have an understanding of this journey through the life course, and to be able to use the theories that describe and explain it in order to organize and enhance your interventions, can only be helpful. This chapter introduces the idea of the life course as an organizing framework for thinking about clients' lives. It presents a number of theoretical ideas and practical tools.

By 'the life course' (Cohler & Hostetler, 2003; Elder *et al.*, 2003), we mean the rhythmic and fluctuating pattern of human life over time, marked out by expected and unexpected life events and interactions between the self and the environment. It covers the journey through life from start to finish, including all the stages, roles and key events that the person experiences, along with the reactions of the person to these experiences and the meanings which they attach to them. To adopt a life course framework is not to adhere to a particular, well-defined theory. Instead, it is to take on a world view or perspective that posits an active and agentic individual interacting with and moving through an influential and modifiable physical and interpersonal environment (McAdams, 1993). The specifics of what this means are spelt out in less abstract terms in Box 1.1, and can be thought of as a manifesto for the life course (or lifespan) perspective. You should look at these statements before reading on, and reflect on the questions posed.

For each and every one of us, the life course is a fascinating and complex personal journey, and for those of us who work therapeutically with others it provides a robust framework that helps divide complicated concepts into smaller, logically related and

13

Box 1.1   A manifesto of the life course perspective

To take a life course perspective towards your work involves adhering to a set of propositions that includes the following assumptions (Baltes, 1987; Rutter, 1989, 1996; Elder, 1996; Elder *et al.*, 2003; Shanahan *et al.*, 2003):

1. People experience both change and continuity throughout their life course.
2. Every person has some unique, some shared and some universal characteristics.
3. Many different factors and dimensions contribute to a person's make-up, and these can change in different ways, at different rates and with different outcomes.
4. All change involves both gains and losses.
5. All change involves the potential, which may or may not be realized, for personal growth.
6. The timing of life events within a person's life course is a significant factor in how those events are perceived and handled.
7. Development and growth arise out of an interaction between the person and his or her environment.
8. The needs of clients are best seen in the context of their physical, interpersonal, cultural and historical situation.

Think about the statements above. They are the viewpoints to which we adhere, but remember that this is what they are: viewpoints, not unambiguous facts or truths.

- Which of the above statements do you agree with most strongly? Why?
- Are there any that you do not agree with? Why?
- Are there any that you do not understand?

We hope that you will understand these tenets better and more fully once you have worked through this text, but for the moment you may like to discuss any uncertainties or confusions with your tutors and/ or colleagues.

more manageable chunks (Pickin & St Leger, 1993). It can be used as an aide-memoire for health and social care professionals' assessment of client needs, and as a tool for the planning and evaluation of interventions.

Roles across the life course

Client-centred intervention includes the belief that meaningful activity both contributes to and is a source of personal well-being; and occupational therapy is specifically grounded in this belief. A life course perspective locates this and, indeed, all activity in the context of one or more social roles, for example the role of worker, parent, student or, possibly for many of your clients, patient. Turn now to Learning Task 1.1, which will help you begin to build up a picture of the lives of the participants in our case study (pp. 6–11).

Learning Task 1.1 Identifying roles

In Learning Task 0.1, you will have completed a genogram that summarizes the ages of the different characters in our case study and the relationships between them. The present activity invites you to begin thinking about these characters in terms of the major roles that they occupy.

By a 'role', we mean those sets of behaviours and attitudes that are associated with particular social positions and that serve a specific function for both individuals and the society of which they are a part.

Below is a list of some of the characters that appear in the case study. Identify their ages and the roles that you know them to occupy. How many of these roles could you have predicted from knowing their age alone?

- Helen
- Richard
- Mary
- Brian
- Sarah
- Chris

Learning Task 1.1 introduces the idea of a person's roles varying across the life course, at least in part dependent on his or her life stage. This can be represented diagrammatically as a *life-career rainbow*. Donald Super (1980; Herr, 1997), the psychologist who introduced this idea, identified nine roles that together are able to account for most of the roles occupied by most people most of the time: *child, student, leisure user, citizen, worker, partner/spouse, homemaker, parent* and *retiree*. Of course, for any particular individual some of these roles may be absent (not everyone is a spouse, for example) or insignificant (there are those for whom studentship comes to an end early in life, has never had much meaning and is never resumed later in life). Similarly, for some people, roles that do not figure in Super's list (for example sibling, client or patient) may be of prime importance. Super identifies four key arenas in which these roles are acted out: home, work, school (or other educational establishment) and community. These are all important parts of the environment or context in which most, although of course not all, individuals live out their lives.

Key issues for occupational therapists and other health and social care practitioners relate to the number, size, nature and personal significance of the constellation of roles that comprise a client's life-career rainbow. Do they represent a good role balance? Are there any significant gaps? Are any roles too demanding for the client? What changes may be indicated in order to further a client's well-being or progress?

The life-career rainbow can indicate more than mere role *occupancy*. Thus, the width of each band can be varied in line with the time demands of a particular role. Immediately after the birth of a first child, parents may find that the 'parent' role occupies almost all hours of the day (and night), with other roles being compressed into small windows of time, or else dropped altogether. After a while, however, the time demands of the role lessen somewhat, and a more balanced and varied role repertoire can be attained. Illness and disability can likewise disrupt a person's role balance, with hitherto important roles being squeezed out of a person's life. As an occupational therapist, you are uniquely placed to address these issues and to work with your clients using the concept of the life-career rainbow to help them to address their needs. It may, in fact, be helpful to spend some time constructing and talking through your client's life-career rainbow quite formally, using the technique of drawing one out as a basis for mutual planning and agreement about goals, aims and interventions. Box 1.2 uses the idea of a life-career rainbow to depict the life course to date of Katie, one of the case study characters.

In thinking about a person's life-career rainbow, it is vital to note that of possibly even greater significance than the time demands of a particular role is its *importance* or *meaning* (or *salience*, to use Super's term). In terms of the life-career rainbow, this could be conveyed by varying the density of the colouring in each band. The colour density of any one role can then vary as the role waxes and wanes in significance. This, even more than the occupancy or not

Box 1.2   Hypothetical life-career rainbow for Katie (adapted from Super, 1980)

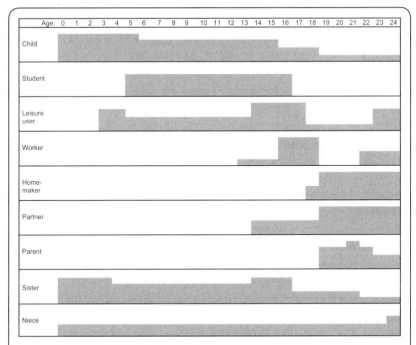

Katie's life-career rainbow is grounded in the information provided in Chapter 0, but it is hypothetical in that it makes assumptions about aspects of her role constellation over time. Nonetheless, it can effectively illustrate how the life-career rainbow can be used to analyse and reflect on issues such as change and stability over time, role balance, role deprivation and role overload. If you look at the list of roles, you will see that the first seven come from Super's list of nine common roles; the roles of *citizen* and *retiree* (or *pensioner*, to use Super's term) have not been included. The remaining two roles, *sister* and *niece*, are not included in Super's list, but are nonetheless identified as significant in Katie's case. The rationale (some aspects more hypothetical than others) for Katie's role occupancy assessments are given below. Note that these comments refer to the time spent in various roles rather than their emotional saliency – that would be something for Katie herself to decide:

- *Child:* This, as for all babies, was the role in which Katie spent most of her infancy and early childhood. In terms of the roles listed above, the only other roles she has occupied since birth are also related to the family, that is the roles of sister and niece. As her world expanded – first into school and work, then into her relationship with Simon and into motherhood – Katie has spent less time in the role of child. It is possible that, in the future, if her parents were to become ill or frail, the child role might again take up a larger part of her life space. She still socializes quite extensively with her mother, Alison, and stepfather, Paul, and so the role remains a significant one for her.

- *Student:* The student role has been a relatively straightforward one for Katie. She started school at the age of five years, and left at the age of 16. Whilst not anti-school, education did not engage her enthusiasm. She left at the earliest opportunity with minimal qualifications, and has no plans to return.

- *Leisure user:* Katie became a leisure user as a child when she joined in pre-school play groups. It continued with her use throughout childhood of the local swimming pool, and took a sudden leap when, as a young teenager, she met Simon and started going 'out on the town'. Since the birth of her sons, Katie's leisure time has been substantially curtailed, although it may be on the rise as her children get older. This might, of course, change if she and Simon have their planned additional children.

- *Worker:* From the age of 12 years, Katie took on a paper round and babysitting jobs, and then worked full-time until the birth of her first son, Ben. For the last couple of years, she has held a part-time job as a care assistant in a local nursing home, working nights to fit in with Simon's work commitments and her childcare responsibilities.

- *Homemaker:* When Katie became pregnant with Ben, she and Simon lived with his parents for a while until they found their own place. This meant that Katie took on some homemaking responsibilities at this time, although these increased significantly, and have remained high, since the family moved into their own house.

- *Partner:* Katie and Simon have been together for ten years, since Katie was 13 years old. The time committed to this relationship increased when Katie became pregnant and she and Simon moved in together.

- *Parent:* The role of mother has been a significant part of Katie's life space ever since the birth of her first son, although, whilst it remains high, the time given to this role has fallen slightly as first Ben and then Dan entered nursery and, in Ben's case, primary school. It is, of course, likely to increase again if she and Simon add to their family.

- *Sister:* Katie has occupied the role of sister since she was born. As a young child, this was a major element in her life space, becoming less central once her elder sister, Sarah, started school. For a few

years in her early teens Katie spent more time socializing with her sister, but this decreased when Sarah began her nursing training, and has remained fairly low ever since.
- *Niece:* Katie has also been a niece for the whole of her life. Since her Aunt Helen's CVA, Katie has voluntarily and markedly increased the time and energy devoted to this role.

of particular roles, can be highly individual and idiosyncratic, making it risky for health and social care workers to make assumptions about the relative significance of a client's various roles. Hence, role saliency is not depicted in the life-career rainbow for Katie. Whilst we may be able to hazard a guess at the saliency for her of some of her roles, at least at some points in her life course, this is really for her to decide. Rather than being assumed, role saliency is something that should be explored with clients as part of the assessment process. The ideal scenario, of course, is when those roles represented by a wide band (that is time-consuming ones) have a good degree of colour density (thereby indicating significant salience to the individual). It may be salutary for us to realize how large a part of a person's life the client role may at times occupy. We need to consider how we can ensure that clients experience our interactions as meaningful as well as time-consuming. Clients, like everyone else, are vulnerable to stress and depression as a consequence of performing roles that occupy a great deal of time but have little salience for them. This is particularly true when those roles last for long periods, and even more so when there appears to be no prospect of things changing.

Now that we have made the case for the value of the life-career rainbow as a way of thinking about the life course, it is time for you to try using it yourself. Learning Task 1.2 asks you to construct your own life-career rainbow. Whilst the main focus of this book, with the exception of the final two chapters, is the client rather than the therapist, it is important to remember that the concepts discussed are applicable to all of us. Furthermore, we are each better placed than anyone else to construct our own life-career rainbow, which is another good reason for asking clients to complete their own with you there rather than you attempting to do it for them.

Learning Task 1.2   Constructing a life-career rainbow

Think of the various roles you have occupied in your life so far, and represent them on a life-career rainbow. Draw the rainbow as a series of horizontal lines, as in Box 1.2, indicating when roles were taken up and when they were dropped. If necessary, include roles not mentioned by Super. Indicate the importance of the roles by variations in the density of shading (the deeper the colour, the more meaningful the role). When you have completed it, ask yourself the following questions about your life-career rainbow and, if possible, discuss your answers with one or more fellow students or colleagues.

- How typical is your life-career rainbow of someone of your age and life stage?
- How is your current situation affecting your constellation of roles?
- How do you imagine your life-career rainbow will change in the future?

Current roles: a snapshot of the 'now'

Whilst the life-career rainbow is a particularly effective tool for monitoring *changes* in role occupancy and significance, a snapshot of a client's *current* role repertoire – in effect, a cross-sectional slice through the life-career rainbow – can more easily be represented in the form of a pie chart. The larger the slice of the 'pie', the greater the time spent in that role. Learning Task 1.3 asks you to complete a pie chart for a client you are, or have been, working with. This can be useful when planning interventions, especially where decisions need to be made about how best your client can spend limited resources of time and energy. As a pre-worked example, we have also included a pie chart of one of the people (Mary) in our case study's current role occupancy. How well balanced do you think her roles seem to be? Are there any that are too great or too small? Which roles does it suggest as being most in need of development or maintenance? How could you, as someone who works with a client-centred approach, try to alter the balance?

During a person's life course, roles exist in an equilibrium that can be affected by illness or disability, and may lead to role imbalance and role underload or deprivation (Creek, 2002), something

Learning Task 1.3   Pie charts to show role occupancy and importance

Here is a pie chart of Mary's current roles. The size of each segment indicates the relative amount of time Mary devotes to each role. Its importance (or emotional salience) is indicated by its shading: black means the role is very important, grey that it is moderately important and white that it is relatively unimportant. In considering Mary's pie chart, do not forget that this is our interpretation of her life, not Mary's. She might divide up the 'pie' somewhat differently, very probably including roles that we know nothing about.

Mary's current key roles

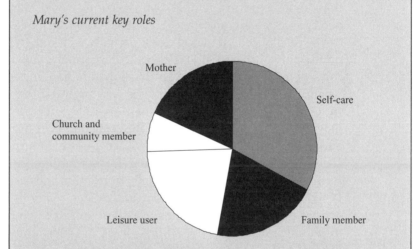

We can see that in this moment-in-time slice through Mary's life-career rainbow our interpretation is that 'Self care' takes up much of her time (being the largest segment) and is reasonably salient to her (being coloured grey). 'Church and community membership' is not currently very meaningful to her, nor does it take up much time. In these examples, time commitment and emotional salience vary in step with each other: self-care is currently both more time-consuming and more important to Mary than is church and community membership. The black colouring of the 'Mother' and 'Family member' sectors indicates that these are what really matter to Mary. The white colouring of the 'Leisure user' sector indicates that it is not an emotionally important occupation for Mary at the moment, although it actually occupies a relatively large amount of her time.

- How would you explain Mary's slice through her life-career rainbow?
- How might you try to modify either her perception of the areas or their size?

Now construct a pie chart to describe the role constellation of a client you are, or have been, working with.

- Add shading to indicate the importance of that role to the client.
- Consider the extent to which 'time commitment' and 'personal significance' match up.

that can lead to considerable distress. For nearly all clients, this area needs assessment, and possibly intervention. It may be that roles can be rebalanced, or even at least partially restored, by skilful work on the part of therapist and client. Alternatively, new occupations, roles or relationships may be developed. Changing the previous balance and pattern of roles may be very important to your clients. In terms of their perception of their own life, such reconfiguration may allow them to perceive both meaning and purpose in daily life, and to find social acceptance. Social acceptance, in turn, means that social support of the role and activity is much more likely to be forthcoming. The holding of socially normative and acceptable roles is likely to enhance self-esteem and foster relationships, giving energy, opportunity and a positive sense of self to your client. The importance of balanced, fulfilling roles in determining quality of life and self-esteem cannot be underestimated.

Recognition of how the client's place in the life course affects role balance is an essential ingredient in planning intervention. As we grow up, we all develop an awareness (although we may not put it into words) of the nature of different life stages. We develop expectations about what we will and/or think we ought to be doing at different points in the life cycle: 'I ought to be financially independent by the time I'm 25', 'I want to be married before I'm 30', 'I expect to be retired at 65', 'I'll need a bungalow or ground-floor flat when I'm 80' are all commonplace examples. The following section provides some theories and concepts for expressing and debating these assumptions.

Stages and developmental tasks across the life course

All societies divide the life course into stages, and these are reflected in the organization of many health and social care services. Sometimes this is explicit, for example paediatric services, adolescent mental health provision, Sure Start programmes for the under-fours or services for older people. Sometimes it is implicit. Thus, services around maternity care, stroke rehabilitation or occupational training will tend to involve clients within a particular life stage because of the association between life stage and a wide range of significant life events. Occupational training, for example, is unlikely to occur with the under-15s or the over-60s. In the past, maternity care was relatively rare in the over-40s, but this has changed latterly and reminds us that what society considers to be the appropriate age for any given role or activity can vary considerably from community to community, society to society and also across different generations. This is, indeed, one of the tenets of the life course perspective's manifesto. Learning Task 1.4 asks you to think about the typical characteristics of different life stages. Give this activity some attention now, before you read on. You may be surprised both by how much you already know about change and development across the life course and by the way in which some life stages are far easier than others to characterize in this way.

Learning Task 1.4   Developmental tasks across the life course

For each of the following age bands, think about what, typically, are the key:

- major life events
- occupational priorities with regard to self-care, productivity and leisure
- personal aspirations and concerns
- social and relationship issues.

Age band:

Birth to 5 years	25–40 years
5–12 years	40–60 years
12–18 years	60–75 years
18–25 years	75+ years

The term 'developmental task' was coined in the 1940s by Robert Havighurst, an American educationalist, who described it as a task that:

arises at or about a certain period in the life of the individual, successful achievement of which leads to . . . happiness and to success with later tasks, while failure leads to unhappiness in the individual, disapproval by the society, and difficulty with later tasks. (Havighurst, 1972, p. 2)

In other words, developmental tasks represent personal developmental milestones and achievements that allow us to progress in society, by easing our way into future tasks and receiving the accolade and approval of those around us. It may be that many of the clients you meet in your professional life are not in a position to conform to these social norms and expectations. They might have been denied many of the day-to-day plaudits that come the way of the majority of the population, and thus may feel that their position in society is tenuous and lacking in value. Arising from this, there may be a sense of powerlessness which will need to be addressed if the person is to make some gains in the quality of their life. It may be necessary to challenge some of the taken-for-granted, normative hallmarks of successful growth and development.

The way in which life events and developmental tasks cluster (or not) around particular points in the life course provides a framework for thinking about life stages that is especially attuned to the goals of most client-centred interventions. Havighurst was interested in the idea of the 'teachable moment': the point or sensitive period in the life course when the person (notably the child) is most receptive to learning a particular skill or type of concept. It is very often the task of the educationalist to identify and exploit this moment. It is not by chance that in many societies formal education begins at the age of five or six years, or that transfer to secondary school occurs between the ages of 11 and 13. These social transitions are timed to coincide with the pattern and nature of most people's cognitive and social development. This can confront the health and social care practitioner with a challenging task. On the one hand, the practitioner wants to facilitate clients' engagement with the tasks with which they would have been engaging, and the attainment as soon and as far as is possible of skills towards which they would have been striving, had they not experienced the life events or circumstances that brought them to the attention of the health and social care professional. On the other hand, this same professional, to a degree that surpasses even that of teachers, is concerned with the uniqueness and individuality of the client. This requires managing the tension between developmental norms and milestones, on the one hand, and the unique competencies and needs of a particular client, on the other. Havighurst's description of developmental tasks as the combined outcome of biological maturation, cultural pressures and individual desires, aspirations and values provides a basis on which occupational therapists and other health and social care practitioners can plan their work with clients.

Because of the involvement of biological and psychological processes that are universal across people, time and place, there will be some commonality of developmental tasks for widely different individuals, families and communities. Because of the involvement of individual differences, varying aspirations, and cultural and social norms in the establishment of developmental tasks, the tasks associated with different life stages will, at the same time, also vary across individuals, cultures and epochs. Thus, whilst Havighurst identified six to nine developmental tasks for each of six age periods, ranging from 'Infancy and early childhood' to 'Later maturity', his recognition of the impact of social, cultural and historical change and difference led him to change and 'update' his list several times during his career. It will, of course, need constant updating and revision long after Havighurst ceases to be in a position to undertake the work, and it will be helpful for those working with it to review it in light of current circumstances and the particular client in question.

Despite variations in the nature and significance of particular developmental tasks, even for people of similar age and background, it is possible to identify some developmental tasks that tend, at least to some extent, to be associated with particular ages and/or life stages. Erikson (1994) identifies a sequence of psychosocial crises or preoccupations that characterize different stages of the life course and which potentially lead to the development of a significant new personal strength. The crises centre on:

- *Trust* (aged 0–1 years): becoming confident that one's basic needs will be met
- *Autonomy* (1–6 years): establishing self-control without loss of self-esteem
- *Purpose* (6–10 years): developing the initiative to strive for goals that will fulfil personal potential
- *Competence* (10–14 years): acquiring the skills needed for full and productive involvement in society

- *Identity* (14–20 years): developing an integrated self-concept and a coherent set of values and beliefs
- *Intimacy* (20–35 years): establishing close, committed relationships with others
- *Generativity* (35–65 years): creating a lasting contribution that will extend beyond one's own lifetime
- *Integrity* (65+ years): becoming acceptant of and satisfied with one's life, and understanding its place as part of a wider humanity.

It is interesting to note that in his own late adulthood Erikson questioned whether the crisis of integrity was in fact the final stage of development. In a posthumously published extension of an earlier work (Erikson, 1997), Erikson's widow and collaborator, Joan, added a new, ninth, developmental stage to the human life course in which, as in the adolescent identity crises, previously resolved crisis points are again confronted. Joan Erikson suggests that, if the daily difficulties which are faced by individuals in their eighties and nineties can be accepted, a path is cleared towards a further developmental stage. This stage is *gerotranscendence* (Tornstam, 1989, 2005): a shift in personal perspective from a materialistic and rational view towards a cosmic and transcendent one.

Whilst it is important to recognize that particular ages and life stages tend to bring with them particular concerns and preoccupations, it is crucial that frameworks such as Erikson's are not seen as a rigid set of inevitable stages. It is best to think of them as a broad backdrop against which a person's specific concerns and preoccupations are played out. Whilst they provide pointers as to the concerns of clients at different life stages (Thomas, 1990), the issues Erikson identifies do not occur only at what he describes as their 'time of special ascendancy'. Issues of trust, identity, intimacy etc. are not resolved once and for all: experience and circumstance may trigger and rekindle them at any time (Jacobs, 1998).

The psychosocial stages identified by Erikson are included in the age-based developmental tasks that are summarized in the left-hand column of Table 1.1, which, despite its length, is illustrative rather than exhaustive. Examine this list and think about how the entries relate to your responses to Learning Task 1.4. Was there a great deal of overlap? What were the differences? Is there anything you would now like to add to your answers? Is there anything you think should be added to the list in Table 1.1?

Table 1.1 Developmental tasks and health issues by life stage (adapted from Havighurst, 1972; Pickin & St Leger, 1993; Rice, 2000; Sugarman, 2001, 2004).

Life stage	Developmental tasks	Some key health issues
Infancy (birth to 2 years)	Social attachment Development of the senses Motor development, leading to walking Learning through sensory and motor interactions with the environment Understanding the nature of objects and the creation of categories Emotional development	Mother's health Quality of pregnancy, delivery and perinatal life Quality of home and immediate external environment Immunization Developmental surveillance Family influences Home accidents
Early childhood: Toddlerhood (2–4 years)	Developing mobility and other physical skills Fantasy play Language development Development of self-control	Family influences Immunization Home accidents Immediate external environment Special needs groups
Early childhood: Early school age (4–6 years)	Sex-role identification Early moral development Sense of self Conceptual skills Group play	Accidents outside the home Formal education and preparation for a healthy lifestyle Peer group influences Special needs groups
Middle childhood (6–12 years)	Friendship Development of concrete thinking Skill learning Self-evaluation Team play	Accidents outside the home Formal education and preparation for a healthy lifestyle Peer group influences Special needs groups Malignancies

Table 1.1 Continued

Life stage	Developmental tasks	Some key health issues
Adolescence (12–18 years)	Physical maturation Development of abstract reasoning Personal ideology Emotional development Membership in the peer group Sexual relationships	Preparation for healthy, independent adult life Accidents outside the home Self-inflicted injury Peer group pressures Risky behaviour (e.g. alcohol and drug use) Sexual activity and contraception Special needs groups
Early adulthood: Emerging adulthood (18–25 years)	Autonomy from parents Gender identity Internalized morality Career choice	Unhealthy lifestyles Accidents, especially road traffic accidents Violence Self-inflicted injury Peer group influences Development of autonomy Risky behaviour (e.g. alcohol and drug use) Homelessness Sexually transmitted diseases, including HIV Contraception and family planning Childbearing Stress Special needs groups
Early adulthood: Young adulthood (25–40 years)	Exploring intimate relationships Childbearing and rearing Work Lifestyle	Unhealthy lifestyles Childbearing and rearing Work-related illness Stress Mental health Health promotion Accidents Malignancies Special needs

Table 1.1   Continued

Life stage	Developmental tasks	Some key health issues
Middle adulthood (40–65 years)	Management of career Renegotiating the couple relationship Expanding caring relationships Management of the household Adjusting to ageing parents Coping with physical changes of ageing	Coronary heart disease Stroke Malignancies Chronic illness Work-related illness Respiratory disease Screening (e.g. for breast cancer and CHD risk factors) Mental health Preparation for later life
Late adulthood: Early-late adulthood (65–75 years)	Promotion of intellectual vigour Redirection of energy toward new roles and activities Acceptance of one's life Development of a point of view about death	Maintenance of function and independence Social isolation Mental health Depression Preparation for later life Acute and chronic illness Disability (particularly impairment of mobility and sensation)
Late adulthood: Late-late adulthood (75+ years)	Coping with physical changes of ageing Development of a psycho-historical perspective Facing the unknown	Maintenance of function Social isolation Quality of housing Acute and chronic illness Multiple morbidity Depression and dementia

You will see that Table 1.1 also includes, in the right-hand column, some health issues and risks that may typically be associated with different life stages. Did the distinguishing features of different life stages that you identified in Learning Task 1.4 include any of these factors?

The developmental tasks associated with different life stages provide us with a ready-made set of personal goals (Reinert, 1980), and normative developmental tasks can help us make decisions about how to order and manage our lives. By the same token, however, such norms can constrain a person's freedom of choice and inhibit people's ability to develop alternative, non-normative lifestyles. This may present particular difficulties for those who are living with illnesses or disability, and those who are socially disaffected. A significant number of the clients you encounter in your professional practice may be unable to achieve some normative developmental tasks. Different stages in the human life course present us with particular opportunities and risks, and many of the clients you meet will have to confront the fact that they are not in step with developmental and age norms. This may cause stress, distress and a sense of not truly belonging to society, even of being cast out or rejected. The effect of this on the client's sense of self-worth may be significant, and much work may need to be done to give the client confidence in the process to be embarked upon. The client may be confronted with a number of unwanted and 'off time' events, and this will almost certainly reduce a person's sense of life satisfaction (Bee & Boyd, 2003). This is the case for several of the people in our case study, and you should turn now to Learning Task 1.5 to consider this further.

Learning Task 1.5 'On time' and 'off time' life events

Part one

This task asks you to consider the interplay between age, gender and developmental tasks.

- Turn back to our case study and the genogram that you completed.
- First of all, make sure that you have included ages in your diagram.
- Now pick out three or four people of different life stages and gender (e.g. Mary, Brian, Katie and Richard).
- From the information you have, what developmental tasks do you think they are currently dealing with?
- What other factors influence their developmental tasks?

If at all possible, compare notes with one or more colleagues or fellow students.

Part two

Now think about other characters in the case study and any 'off time' life events they are experiencing. You would probably include in your list:

- Helen's experience of her stroke that, to her, is symbolic of being old (she is no longer able to drive and has lost a significant amount of her capacity for self-care).
- Richard's need to cope, at age 18, with his mother's serious illness.

What other examples of 'off time' events can you identify?

Consider, ideally in discussion with one or more colleagues, why the experience of 'off time' events may present particular challenges.

A quick recap

Already in this chapter we have introduced a number of key concepts that are useful for understanding clients from a life course, or lifespan, perspective. You should, by now, have some understanding of:

- what is meant by the term 'life course', and what it means to adopt a life course perspective
- life roles, and the associated ideas of role overload, role underload and role balance
- the life-career rainbow and pie charts as ways of representing and exploring life roles
- life stages, and their associated developmental tasks
- the tension between shared or normative experiences across the life course and individual uniqueness.

If you are unclear about any of these concepts, have another look through this chapter. You could also consult the section *Key Terms and Concepts*, which you will find towards the end of the book (p. 177). This aims to provide definitions for most of the terms and ideas used in this text. It is important that you have a clear sense of the ideas put forward so far: without them, the remainder of the text is likely to be more than a little confusing.

There are two other general concepts that will help you to make sense of the remainder of this text, to use the ideas it contains in your day-to-day work as a health and social care professional and to enhance your theoretical understanding of the enterprise in which you are engaged. The first concept is the idea of the individual as occupying a particular contextual, or ecological, niche, and the second is the notion of generic developmental tasks that are implicated at all stages of the life course.

Ecological niche

A major element of life course theory as it applies to therapeutic practice is the need to consider and understand clients in their personal, social, cultural and generational context. The theoretically best of plans will come to nothing if no consideration is given to the feasibility of a client translating good intentions into actions. It is necessary to look beyond individual clients to the context and circumstances in which they live their lives; and a way of doing this is to focus not merely on the self, or the person, of the client but on a broader concept that can be variably described as their 'life space' (Peavy, 2004), their 'personal niche' (Willi, 1999) or their 'life structure' (Levinson, 1990). This includes their family and wider social and cultural circumstances. The life space, or life structure, as the core focus of attention for the occupational therapist is discussed in Chapter 2. For the present, we want you to think of the client as occupying a particular ecological niche (Bronfenbrenner, 1994) at the centre of a concentric circle of influences and environments. It is as if the person is the pip at the centre of an apple, or the softest, innermost heart of an onion – in sum, the centre of a series of nested environments that exert a range of close to distant influences. The ecological view of the person can be captured diagrammatically, as shown in Box 1.3. It is a model that describes the environmental influences on a client, ranging from very specific, concrete factors that impinge directly and immediately on the person to very broad cultural influences.

At the most immediate level, the *settings*, or microsystems, are the everyday environments or arenas in which the person operates. These arenas can encompass home, school, work, neighbourhood and, for clients such as Helen in our case study, hospital. They include relationships with, for example, spouse, children, friends, employers, colleagues and, again for clients such as Helen, many different health and social care professionals and voluntary agencies. Questions relating to parenthood (for example 'How does Helen's illness affect the lives of Andrew and Richard?') or the volunteer role ('How may Helen feel about losing contact with the

Box 1.3   An ecological view of the person (adapted from Bronfenbrenner, 1994)

Bronfenbrenner embeds the person in a series of environmental forces that range from being very close and immediate to being very broad and general. These can be represented visually as a series of concentric circles, as shown below:

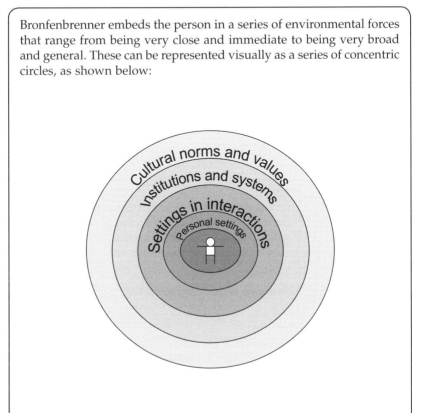

If you turn back to Chapter 0 and the paragraph about nine-year-old Chris (p. 10), you will see that some of the contextual influences that impinge on him include:

- *Personal settings*
  - ○ home and immediate family (Alison and Paul)
  - ○ extended family (Sarah and Ranjiv, Katie and Simon, Ben, Dan, grandparents, Wicket the dog)
  - ○ school and school friends
  - ○ family friends
  - ○ football team
  - ○ athletics club
  - ○ leisure club
  - ○ neighbours and neighbourhood
- *Settings in interactions*
  - ○ friends from school who also play football or go running
  - ○ friends from school who are neighbours

- relatives who attend his school
- adults who look after him at home and facilitate his different activities away from home
- adults who are concerned with his home, school, neighbourhood and activities
- loyalties to different parts of the family
- *Institutions and systems*
  - local education authority
  - city and county council
  - the broader governmental and political agenda (including education, health, child benefit etc.)
- *Cultural norms and values*
  - beliefs about the importance of family, school and community
  - religious beliefs (several family members are active in the church)
  - cultural views and expectations (including the perceived importance of sporting prowess, assumptions about family members' futures, friendships, future activities and aspirations)
  - views on illness and death

Think about the influence of all these different factors on Chris, the person he is and is likely to become.

housebound parishioners that she has visited regularly for several years?') clearly relate to the concepts included in the idea of ecological niche and are the sort of thing that the practitioner may need to explore with Helen.

Interactions between settings occur when different microsystems overlap: home and hospital, work and home, or work and community, for example. Here, questions for Helen may include how to fit in social contacts around hospital appointments (community and home) or how to access practical resources that will enable her to continue her keen interest in gardening (home and leisure).

The next level is that of *institutions and systems* rather than individual organizations: prevalent economic policy, health authorities, education authorities, for example, rather than particular hospitals, schools, voluntary services etc. The type of issue to be explored here includes the indirect impact of those institutions on the person. How, for example, will the local bus and train timetables (a reflection of national and local transport policy) affect Helen's social opportunities or the accessibility of various community services? Similarly, the relationship between the various services which Helen may need will have an impact on how her recovery and quality of life are managed. Such issues are embedded in the local and national institutions and systems surrounding Helen's life.

At the broadest level of influence are *cultural norms and values*. These consist of general cultural expectations, such as predominant beliefs and ideologies and notions of the normal, expectable life course. How, for example, will Helen feel about not being able to work, at least for the time being, at an age when work is often an important part of life? Will she be concerned about being 'non-productive' in a society where independence, achievement and autonomy are all highly valued?

Chapter 2 explores in detail the use of a self-in-context perspective for planning and implementing work with clients.

Generic developmental tasks

Thinking about age and/or life stage focuses attention on the ways in which developmental tasks change across the life course, bringing into the spotlight the distinguishing features of each phase of life. It is important for anyone working in a client-centred framework to take these into account in order to ensure that clients' treatment programmes are appropriate for their age, life stage and lifestyle, and are focused specifically on that individual client.

In addition, the life course perspective normalizes the experience of change across the whole of the life span. It identifies a number of broad developmental tasks that are common to all life stages, highlighting the fact that we face many similar challenges at various points in the life course, and that we have developed, and can continue to develop, strategies for managing these challenges that are transferable across both tasks and stages. These generic developmental tasks provide the structure for Chapters 3–6. They include coping with life events (Chapter 3), dealing with transitions and loss (Chapter 4), managing stress (Chapter 5) and decision-making and problem-solving (Chapter 6). When clients talk about their lives, they do not generally structure their accounts neatly around theoretical concepts such as life events, transitions and stress. Rather, clients weave their accounts into a narrative and present themselves to therapists through the stories they tell. That their story is in some way problematic or awry is what brings clients into the care of occupational therapists and other health and social care professionals (Howard, 1991). Healing and treatment can then be seen as a process of story repair and (re)construction. This narrative perspective is considered in Chapter 7.

The person of the therapist

After this consideration of ecological niche, generic developmental tasks and personal narrative, it is, in our final two chapters, the experience of the health and social care professional, specifically the experience of being an occupational therapist, that takes centre stage. Chapter 8 is based on a study of the life-career experiences of occupational therapists who move from practice into occupational therapy education (Wright, 2007) and focuses on the process of being and belonging as a member of the occupational therapy professional community. Chapter 9 strives to bring all the threads of our arguments together and consider their significance for both your initial training and your continuing professional development.

Armed with a secure understanding of the concepts introduced in this chapter, you are well placed to work with your clients from a life course perspective and take a client-centred view of your intervention plan within a holistic framework. We believe this will equip you to work creatively with clients of various ages and at different life stages, who present with various challenges and difficulties, and to work with those involved with them, be they family, friends, colleagues, informal carers or other health and social care professionals. The remaining chapters in this text will provide you with a more detailed understanding of these issues. Like the life course itself, we hope you will find this text a journey of discovery.

2. *The Client in Context*

When working as a health or social care professional, it is important to work as holistically as possible. Clients need to be seen as whole people, not as bundles of disembodied symptoms or problems. Their entire beings and the contexts in which their lives are played out must be taken into account and respected if intervention is to be both useful and respectful. The acknowledgement of the significance of context for individuals means that the developmental tasks that form the basis of Chapters 3 through to 6 are broad ranging, extending far wider than specifically health- – or even well-being – related issues. Beyond this, we recognize that we each live in a shared space that is not ours alone to change. This is the essence of the ecological view of the person introduced in Chapter 1. It embraces as fundamental the assumption that the interpersonal, social and cultural contexts in which clients live their lives cannot be ignored; indeed, their influence is profound at every level and at every stage. The present chapter focuses on ways of capturing this idea of client-in-context. It supplements the concept of the self with that of the personal life space (Peavy, 2004) or niche (Willi, 1999) – people and the segment of the social, cultural and material environment that is meaningful to them and with which they interact. Peavy (2004) describes the life space as being made up of experiences, meanings, objects, activities, interactions and the solitude of being alone. It includes all the internal and external forces that influence the person at any moment, and, whilst each person's life space is unique, Peavy identifies five broad life space 'sectors':

- world view, perspective, values, personal philosophy of life, spirituality
- intimate relationships, family, friends, love

- health, illness, well-being, body image, physical functioning
- work, training, employment, unemployment, education
- play, leisure, recreation, creativity, personal renewal.

These sectors are linked by the voice of the self, and reinforce the belief, first penned as early as the seventeenth century, that 'No man is an island'. Of course, we would now add 'and neither are women and children'! Its holistic emphasis means that your work as an occupational therapist may roam over any or all sectors of a client's life space.

Life space mapping

One way that we can usefully explore the personal life space is through the process of mapping (Peavy, 2004; Rodger, 2006), taking, in effect, a cross-sectional slice through the life-career rainbow and extending the pie charts you completed in Learning Task 1.3 (p. 21). Life space mapping offers a useful additional approach in that it cuts across the various roles people fulfil and allows them to put together the different elements of their life in the way they choose, rather than imposing a particular (in this case, role-based) structure.

As with both the life-career rainbow and the pie chart, it is not merely the content of the personal life space that is important. Of even greater significance is the personal meaning of its elements and the relationships between them. A personal life space contains all those meanings (of people, experiences, belongings, relationships, events and so on) that a person has accumulated in life so far. In our professional lives, we are continually engaging with clients in an investigation of their life space in order to empower, enhance or restore how they experience their current state and their future. Life space mapping (see Learning Task 2.1) is a way of doing this explicitly. Working from the notion that a picture tells a thousand words, it invites participants to draw a map that indicates visually the importance of certain features of their lives, as well as the relationships between these different elements. One useful aspect of drawing this type of map is that it is accessible to clients who do not find the written word, or even the spoken word, the best or most useful way of expressing their ideas. It provides a potentially non-verbal and less structured way of describing the life space. More creative, perhaps unacknowledged, or even new, ideas

Learning Task 2.1   Life space mapping

Below is a hypothetical life space map for Paul, who, as Helen's brother-in-law, is seemingly one of the more peripheral characters in our case study. However, the close relationship between his son, Chris, and Helen may lead to Paul's greater involvement in the implications of Helen's CVA. What you see below is a life space map created from the limited information available about Paul in Chapter 0, plus a few speculations. Whilst such a map may be a valuable starting point for health and social care professionals when working with a particular client, it should be remembered that, ideally, in keeping with client-centred practice, life space maps should be constructed by the clients themselves.

In this life space map, we see Paul placed like a sun at the centre of a solar system. The positioning of the other elements in the map gives some indication of their relationship to Paul and to each other. The central elements in Paul's life are shown to be his wife, Alison, and son, Chris. Indeed, the relationship between these three is seen as so close that the elements are overlapping. Because of this closeness, elements in the map to which Paul relates only indirectly – including Alison's mother (Helen) and other members of her family – are also a part of Paul's life space. Paul's family (parents, siblings and cousins) are, after Alison and Chris, the people with the most central role in his life. He also, however, is shown as having a direct relationship with Alison's two daughters, Katie and Sarah, and their partners. Sarah and Rajiv's location on the map, being further away from Paul than Katie and her family, suggests that Paul feels more distant from them, possibly seeing less of them and feeling that they have fewer shared interests and values.

Although personal relationships dominate Paul's life space map, other elements are included. Closest to him is the element of 'Pubs and clubs', which denotes the site of his and Alison's social life. This element includes the places – the pubs and clubs themselves – but also the relationships and activities that occur there. Note, also, how the line linking 'Pubs and clubs' with Paul's extended family suggests their connection with these places as well. Two other boxes indicate employment-related activities as a part of Paul's life space. Mediated through Alison herself is Alison's part-time job in a local shop. Although the job itself does not impinge on Paul, it may be a significant element in his life space because of the need to arrange child care and other commitments around its demands. As their only regular source of earned income, it is likely to play an important role financially as well. Paul's own work is placed right at the edge of his map – suggesting its subsidiary role in his life. The broken line linking 'Paul' to 'work' further hints at his tenuous involvement with paid employment.

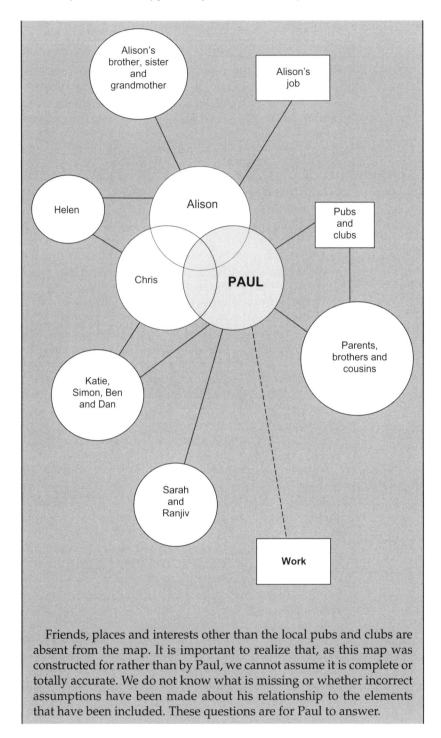

Friends, places and interests other than the local pubs and clubs are absent from the map. It is important to realize that, as this map was constructed for rather than by Paul, we cannot assume it is complete or totally accurate. We do not know what is missing or whether incorrect assumptions have been made about his relationship to the elements that have been included. These questions are for Paul to answer.

Your task

Your task is to construct a picture of your own personal life space through the technique of life space mapping. Whilst it is perfectly possible to do this task on your own, it will be more interesting and informative if you could then discuss your map in pairs or a small group since you are all likely to have tackled the task somewhat differently. Discuss and talk through how you constructed your map, and what the significance of the different elements is.

For this task you will need, at a minimum, a large sheet of paper (at least A3 size) and some felt-tip pens, ideally of various sizes and colours. Your life space map could possibly be squashed onto a sheet of your Learning Journal, but you will able to be more creative and comprehensive if you give yourself a larger canvas to work on.

It can also be very useful to arm yourself with a number of small Post-it notes. This means you can use one Post-it note for each element within your life space, moving them around on the map until you are satisfied with their location. If you use Post-it notes of different colours, you can colour code the elements if you like, one colour for each type of element.

Use these materials to construct a 'map' that depicts the people, activities, plans and other elements that are important parts of your life at the current time.

Whilst there are many ways to construct a life space map – and, certainly, there are no right or wrong ways – we suggest the following procedure:

- Take your sheet of paper and place your name in the centre of the page.
- Write each significant element in your personal life space – particular people, events, experiences, objects etc. – on a separate Post-it note.
- Show the importance of these elements to you and to each other through the physical placement of the elements on the map. Move the elements around until you are satisfied with their placement.
- Use connecting lines, drawings, words, colours and shading etc. to indicate the quality and nature of the interrelationships between the elements and between them and you.
- When complete, reflect on the nature of your life space. How happy are you with it? What are its strengths and weaknesses? How rich a tapestry is it? What is missing? What would you like to change?

may emerge. These ideas can initiate new trains of thought that may be helpful in the planning of interventions that take the client's life forward in progressive and innovative ways, and that meet needs in an individualized and effective manner.

Even though clients may find constructing a life space map intrinsically interesting (provided it does not trigger too many anxieties about their drawing skills), it is a means to an end rather than an end in itself. It is what emerges from the exercise that is most important. Useful questions to ask of a life space map include:

- How do you feel about your life space map? How accurate, complete and satisfactory is it?
- What type of item is included in the map? Is it mainly other people, or does it include elements such activities, places, belongings, organizations or personal values?
- Are the items positive and facilitative or negative and inhibitory – or both?
- What is the direction of impact? The person on the elements? The elements on the person? Both?
- If you suddenly had the power to do so, what would be the main thing you would change about your life space? What difference would this make?
- How has the map changed? What might it have looked like six months, two years or even ten years ago?
- How may it change in the future? How would you *like* it to change in the future?

The relationships between the different parts of the map indicate how individuals make meaning of their world. Reflection on the map and dialogue between client and therapist about the map can help to clarify or reveal personal values, assumptions and opinions that the client might not have previously put into words. A person's life space is dynamic and changing, and comparing past and present life space maps can be a useful way of exploring change and loss. Think about Richard, the younger son of Helen Case. In the immediate aftermath of his mother's CVA, his life space would have been very different from how it had been previously. His imagined map of the future would, likewise, have been similarly disrupted, although, with time, he may re-introduce some of his previous hopes, plans and aspirations.

Life space mapping can be very useful when imagining and planning for the future (Shepherd, 1999). From maps of hoped-for selves, specific scripts, plans and action strategies can be developed to promote movement towards them. Similarly, concrete actions can be taken to avoid or come to terms with feared future selves. Furthermore, the work involved in life space mapping may include several other skills or activities that are relevant for a particular client; these include conversational and concentration skills, creative thinking and fine-motor coordination, organizational skills or the ability to think about the present and the future. As the map can be seen as a snapshot of a person's world view at a particular point in time, keeping the map (or taking a photograph or photocopy of it) and repeating the exercise at a later date can provide a basis for exploring and monitoring change over time (Rodger, 2006).

Stability zones: anchors in the personal life space

Many clients of health and social care professionals will have suffered a trauma that severely disrupts the stability and tranquillity of their personal life space. Their sense of identity and security, as well as their self-esteem and confidence, are very likely to have been disturbed. Helen is the clearest example of this from the case study (p. 7). Her unexpected and untimely stroke will almost certainly mean that her independence, her confidence in her own health, her roles as mother, carer for her mother, teacher and church visitor have all taken a severe battering. This is very likely to have had a significant effect on her view of herself, her self-confidence and her sense of security. In situations such as Helen's, elements within the life space that have not been lost or turned upside down assume enhanced significance. They operate as anchors, or stability zones (Open University, 1992; Pedler *et al.*, 2006), that we depend on when all else is confused, uncertain and frightening. Interventions in these circumstances may usefully include the development of new stability zones and the strengthening of those that remain.

More or less, any element within the personal life space has the potential to operate as a stability zone. Frequently, however, they are associated with *people*, *activities*, *ideas and values*, *places*, *belongings* and *organizations*.

- *People* stability zones are sources of social support. They represent valued and enduring relationships with others, for example family members, long-standing friends and colleagues. An important question for you to reflect on is the role of the occupational therapist as a stability zone for clients. Your role may be neither long-standing nor enduring and it is important that you consider the implications of this.

- *Activities* that operate as stability zones (for example hobbies or sport) offer support or distraction. These are a crucial part of every life, as people are essentially active, occupational beings. Trauma, disability and illness can disrupt activity-based stability zones, and it can be an important role for occupational therapists to work with clients to address the implications of this.

- *Ideas and values* that are stability zones underpin our personal standards and philosophy about the meaning of life. They may take the form of deeply held religious beliefs, or strong personal commitments to a philosophy, profession, political ideology or cause. A significant part of your training is concerned with elaborating on, exploring and encouraging you to engage with the ideas and values underpinning occupational therapy practice. Perhaps key tenets of this particular profession – for example belief in the enhancement of well-being through promoting independence or social contact – are already a part of your 'ideas and values' stability zone repertoire.

- *Places* of varying scale can comprise stability zones. They can be large scale (like a country) or small scale (for example a street or a particular room). 'Home' is often a stability zone, a place with a comforting familiarity about it, perhaps where someone grew up or has spent considerable time. When clients are discharged after a long stay in hospital or when a rehabilitation programme at a day centre comes to an end, it may be important to remember that, along with any gains achieved in terms of steps towards independence and well-being, they may be losing contact with a place that has become a significant stability zone for them. It is important for you to establish ways in which your clients can be supported in managing such losses.

- *Belongings* as stability zones take the form of favourite, familiar or comforting possessions. They can range from family heirlooms and particular objects to favourite items of clothing. Bringing mementoes of home and loved ones into hospital or residential care of any kind, for example, can help clients maintain a link with their other stability zones, helping them feel more secure and less disoriented. Think about situations in which you have been away from your home, perhaps when you moved away to college or university, had a spell in hospital or went on an overnight trip with school. Were there any items of sentimental value that you missed or took with you? To what extent can you identify these objects as stability zones?

- *Organizations* that you belong to can act as stability zones. They may include professional bodies, work organizations, social clubs or any other organization to which you belong and with which you identify. Depending on the stage you are at in your career, your organizational stability zones can include your training institution, the professional body or the organization for which you work. There will, of course, be others not related to professional life. Some of your clients may identify with organizations as stability zones which may seem quite alien to you, but it is important not to underestimate the potential worth of such affiliations. It is also important to be aware of our own stability zones so that you do not confuse yours with those of your clients.

It will be clear from some of the above examples that stability zones may overlap: 'home' has elements of place, people and belongings, for example, 'books' have elements of things and ideas and 'the workplace' may have elements of all stability zones. As computers, and especially the Internet, take on an increasingly significant role in many people's lives – as sources of information and activities and, in particular, as gateways to social networks (Boyd & Ellison, 2007) – they represent a potentially important stability zone for many people. Clients whose condition restricts their mobility or capacity for verbal interaction may be able to develop new stability zones through Internet use. However, whilst this may provide purposeful activity and valuable contacts, it is important to consider what could be the downside, or disadvantages, of such a strategy in, for example, exacerbating a client's isolation from face-to-face interactions (Kraut *et al.*, 1998, 2002). There also may be significant safety and privacy concerns, especially in relation to potentially vulnerable clients.

The concept of stability zones can provide a valuable lens through which to explore a person's life space map. You may, for example, ask:

- How adequate is someone's repertoire of stability zones?
- What should be retained and what needs changing?
- Have some elements outlived their usefulness?
- Are there any gaps?
- How enduring are the person's stability zones likely to be?

Turn now to Learning Task 2.2, which invites you to explore the concept of stability zones by searching for examples within the case study.

Learning Task 2.2   Stability zones

- From the case study find examples of the different types of stability zone:
  - people
  - places
  - activities
  - belongings
  - ideas and values
  - organizations
- Who in the case study do you think has the most impoverished collection of stability zones? Who has the richest? What may be the implication of this for their well-being?
- What about your stability zones? Can you identify them? How effective and resilient are they? Do they need attention?

Stability zones can never be sorted out once and for all. Needs, situations and roles change with time and life stage. Belongings wear out, activities may no longer be possible or engaging, houses become too big or too small, friends and colleagues move on, organizations and places change, other people have their own lives to follow and ideas are found to be outmoded or deficient. Similarly, a person's requirements of his or her stability zones will also evolve over time. They need, therefore, regular clarification and nurturing: time needs to be given to maintaining a balance of stability zones so that some are always available to provide reassurance, security and confidence if others are lost.

The personal life space in a life course context

A life space map is like a snapshot, capturing a picture of the person at a particular point in time. Life space maps that are completed either to recall a previous personal life space or to anticipate a future one recognize the dynamic and changing nature of the life course. Awareness that stability zones may need developing and updating similarly acknowledges that both people and environments change over time. In other words, the personal life space needs to be seen in a life course context. If we think of the a life space map as a slice through a tube, we can envisage the person as at the centre of a network of elements that act as a life course convoy (Kahn & Antonucci, 1980, 1981; Antonucci & Akiyama, 1994, 1995), supporting and transporting the person through life. Learning Task 2.3 illustrates this idea visually, and invites you to reflect on your own personal life space and social support convoy across time.

Learning Task 2.3 The life course as a convoy

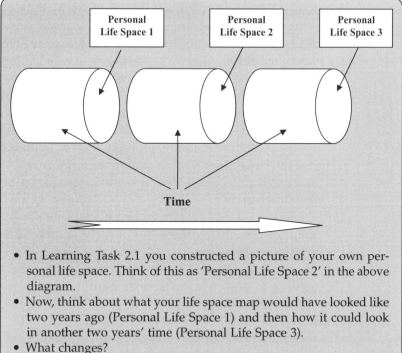

- In Learning Task 2.1 you constructed a picture of your own personal life space. Think of this as 'Personal Life Space 2' in the above diagram.
- Now, think about what your life space map would have looked like two years ago (Personal Life Space 1) and then how it could look in another two years' time (Personal Life Space 3).
- What changes?
- What remains the same?
- Who or what supported you through these changes?

The idea of the life course convoy exemplifies the first point in the manifesto of the life course perspective proposed in Chapter 1, namely that people experience both change and continuity throughout their life course. We now consider the two elements of this proposition in a little more detail.

Change in the personal life space

Change and development do not occur either randomly or evenly across the life course. The notion of life stages, with boundaries (albeit sometimes rather vague and fuzzy ones) between them, suggests a pattern of change that involves periods of significant turmoil and upheaval (as in the adage 'It never rains, but it pours' or 'Troubles always come in threes'), interspersed with periods of greater stability and incremental change (as in 'A step at a time' or 'Slow, but steady'). This pattern is enshrined in Daniel Levinson's model of the life course as the evolution of the personal life space (or 'life structure', to use Levinson's term) through a sequence of alternating periods of change and consolidation (Levinson *et al.*, 1978; Levinson, 1986). Within early and middle adulthood, Levinson (1986) identifies:

- *Early Adult Transition* (from age 17 to 22 years): a developmental bridge between pre-adulthood and early adulthood.
- *Entry Life Structure for Early Adulthood* (22 to 28 years): a time for building and maintaining an initial way of living as an adult.
- *Age 30 Transition* (28 to 33 years): an opportunity to reappraise and modify the entry structure and create the basis for the next life structure.
- *Culminating Life Structure for Early Adulthood* (33 to 40 years): a time for completing the tasks of early adulthood and realizing youthful aspirations.
- *Midlife Transition* (40 to 45 years): a major period of upheaval serving to both terminate early adulthood and initiate middle adulthood.
- *Entry Life Structure for Middle Adulthood* (45 to 50 years): a time for establishing an initial basis for life in middle adulthood.
- *Age 50 Transition* (50 to 55 years): an opportunity for modifying and perhaps improving the entry life structure of middle adulthood.

- *Culminating Life Structure for Middle Adulthood* (55 to 60 years): a time for consolidating and concluding the mid-life era.
- *Late Adult Transition* (60 to 65 years): a boundary period between middle and late adulthood, separating and linking these two eras.

First proposed during the late 1970s, Levinson's model of the life course played a major role in challenging the frequently unarticulated assumption that the years of adulthood normally comprise a relatively uneventful plateau. Instead of this, the model proposes periods of change, typically lasting between three and five years, followed by consolidation periods of about five to seven years. During the periods of change or transition, key elements of the personal life space are transformed in nature and/or significance. Some elements may be lost altogether – as when roles identified in the life-career rainbow are dropped, for example when leaving education and therefore ceasing to have a student role. By the same token, new elements may be introduced, such that, by the end of the period of change, the structure of the personal life space differs considerably from how it had been previously. During the period of consolidation that follows, the detail of the personal life space may be refined, and there may be development and change within its elements, but there is far less change in roles or priorities than that which occurs during the periods of transition. In short, the personal life space has a more settled quality. However, with time, an accumulation of pressure for change builds up within the individual and within the environment, so that the person is eventually propelled into a further period of upheaval, and a new transitional phase begins. In Learning Task 2.4, you can consider these ideas in relation to characters from the case study.

Learning Task 2.4   The evolving life structure

Part one

- Look through the genogram that you constructed for the Case family and allocate each of them to their life stage according to Levinson's (1986) model.
- Look more closely at the life structure of Sarah. At age 24, Sarah (according to Levinson) is likely to be in a structure building phase,

consolidating her Entry Life Structure for Early Adulthood. To what extent and in what ways is, or is not, this the case?

- Now turn your attention to Alison. At age 43, Levinson would place her in the midst of the Midlife Transition. To what extent and in what ways does this seem compatible with her current concerns and roles?
- What impact, if any, has Helen's illness had on the personal life space of Sarah and Alison?

Part two

- Think about your own life course or the life course of friends or family members.
- To what extent can you identify a pattern of alternating periods of change and stability?
- What triggered the periods of change? Was it factors internal to the individual, demands from the environment or a combination of both?
- How stable are the periods of consolidation? What issues triggered the next transitional phase?

It should, of course, be clear that the periods of consolidation are not devoid of change. It is rather that the change is of a more gradual, incremental nature, growing out of elements within the life space rather than dramatically changing them. In other words, there is change within the continuity. By the same token, the periods of change and transition are not totally devoid of continuity. We emerge substantially, but not completely, different. In this way, we are able to maintain a continuous sense of who we are, and explain our current behaviour and aspirations as in some way connected to what has come before. Much life course theory, however, and, indeed, much professional practice in health and social care, is concerned with change, and it is sometimes easy to overlook the significance of continuity. Whilst the concept of stability zones is a good counter to this tendency, it is also worth giving the issue of continuity across the life course further consideration.

Continuity in the personal life space

Personal continuity in our sense of self and in our environment is achieved when we apply familiar strategies in familiar arenas of life

(Atchley, 1999). The continuity that we are talking about here is dynamic rather than static. Whereas static continuity implies something that is unchanging, dynamic continuity enshrines the idea of basic structures which persist over time, but which allow for a variety of changes to occur within the context provided by that structure. The structures that persist over time can be both within the external environment and within the internal disposition of the person, enabling us to distinguish between external and internal continuity. External continuity is achieved by being in familiar environments, undertaking familiar activities and skills, and interacting with familiar people. Internal continuity involves maintaining a consistent sense of who we are – of self and identity. It involves our awareness of the persistence of our personal qualities such as temperament, affect, values, preferences and skills.

Both external and internal continuities may, however, be threatened, and, of the two, it is external continuities that are the more vulnerable. External continuities may be disrupted by such factors as role changes, geographical relocation, depletion of social support networks and changes in health status. Thus, Helen Case has experienced significant external discontinuity: her role as an infant-school teacher has been lost and it is not yet clear whether it is one that she will be able to return to, for example. It is worth reflecting on the extent to which your clients may have lost external continuities, and noting the lack of the familiar in their current situation. Your work environment, which may well contribute to your own sense of external continuity, is likely to be very remote from the experience of many clients. They will, however, be deeply attached to their own environments, which will probably be entirely unfamiliar to you. When these are threatened or disrupted, this can have a negative effect on affect and functioning. Note how, in the case study, several of the characters hesitated and faltered when the ramifications of Helen's illness forced them into confronting strange and unknown situations.

Whilst disruptions to external continuity can threaten our sense of self-consistency, cohesiveness and identity, it is often the case that such upheavals can be incorporated into our personal life space in a way that preserves our sense of inner continuity. Despite our experience of external discontinuity, internally we may be able to see ourselves as much the same person as we always were. Thus, if we retire from work, for example, we might retain our professional identity, seeing ourselves as essentially still belonging to that community of practice, perhaps by joining a group for retired members, making an effort to keep abreast of professional issues or maintaining contact with old colleagues. Even if we feel that we have changed significantly, we will almost always look to events or experiences in our past to 'explain' and make sense of these changes – thus reassuring ourselves of our essential stability and continuity.

Some experiences, however, so disrupt our sense of internal continuity that we are forced to reorganize substantially our definition of 'who we are'. It may be easier for Helen to adjust to the loss of her role as a school teacher than to accept that, rather than being 'the sort of person' who helps others (through her church visiting, for example) she is now 'the sort of person' who receives such support from others. These crises of identity can be, and indeed usually are, disconcerting and distressing. This is likely to be what a number of your clients are experiencing – especially, perhaps, those facing conditions with serious but uncertain outcomes, such as dementia, AIDS, multiple sclerosis or cancer. Lacking a perception of continuity makes a person's life seem unpredictable and chaotic. This can engender a sense of powerlessness. If extreme, this lack of perception of continuity can destroy mental health. Severe discontinuity means that we have no standard against which to assess our life's integrity. The result can be severe anxiety and depression, a lack of hope born of the inability to predict one's future with any confidence. Thus, conditions that affect memory, such as amnesia and Alzheimer's disease, may lead those who have these conditions to no longer know who they are or were, to not know who the other characters in their life story are or even what the plot of the story may be.

However, it is also important to remember that the life course perspective adopts a 'developmental' rather than a 'pathological' attitude towards change – as noted in Point 5 of the manifesto of the life course perspective: all change involves the potential for personal growth. Whilst being aware of the risks to well-being that accompany disruptions to our life space, working from a life course perspective involves, as Woolfe (2001) reminds us, adopting a mindset in which:

> crises are perceived as normative human experiences that pose a challenge and an opportunity for developmental adaptation and growth. An emphasis is placed on well-being rather than

sickness, and in understanding individuals' problems within a
social and cultural matrix. (Woolfe, 2001, p. 347)

So, we must recognize that not all threats to either internal or external continuity are undesirable or unwelcome. Indeed, many appear as positive, anticipated and/or 'natural' stages or phases of the life course. The development of our species, in fact, is predicated on a positive response to change and the seeking of it as we strive to maintain our survival and improve our conditions. We seek a balance between a sense of sameness on the one hand and challenge on the other. Some elements of the familiar we may be pleased to lose, and whilst external continuity can be seen by others, it is only the individuals themselves who can ascribe meaning to the experience of continuity or change. Furthermore, people differ in the extent to which they see the search for novelty or change as important, and the extent to which this experience of change is believed to be desirable. Thus, the degree of continuity attributed by individuals to their lives can be classified as too little, too much or optimum. If people experience too little continuity, life seems uncomfortably unpredictable. If they experience too much, life seems dull and routine. Optimum continuity is that where individuals see the pace and degree of change as being in line with their coping capacity. It is where they experience their lives as sufficiently challenging to dispel any sense of boredom or stagnation; but not so challenging as to be overwhelming. As health and social care professionals, you will frequently be engaged in working with clients to find this constantly changing point of balance between change and continuity.

3.   *Life Events*

Everybody, everywhere, whatever their life stage, is experiencing life events of some sort. Most people are experiencing several. Take some time now to use Learning Task 3.1 as a vehicle for thinking about your own current and recent life events.

Learning Task 3.1   My current life events

It is very easy to talk about significant life events in our own and our clients' lives without really thinking about what we mean by the term and, very importantly, whether we all mean the same thing. This task is designed to encourage you to think about the nature and range of significant life events and factors influencing how, and how well, they are managed. This time, you are asked to think about your own life events rather than those of a client or a member of the Case family.

First, make a list of the key life events you have experienced during the last 24 months. Give yourself a bit of time to think about this: don't stop as soon as you come to an initial pause. It may be that, on reflection, events that seemed trivial at the time in retrospect can be identified as 'significant'.

When your list is complete (although you can, of course, add to it later), ask yourself, and make notes on, the following questions about the events on your list:

- How would I describe the event? What were its key characteristics?
- What personal resources did I use to handle it?
- Who helped or supported me? Who hindered me?
- What did I actually do? What coping skills did I use?

Life events vary along a number of key dimensions. Some are planned; others not. Some are welcomed; others not. All life events require coping strategies to manage the changed circumstances. This applies whether the events are perceived as good (for example a pay rise, a job, a new baby or finishing the final piece of course work) or bad (divorce, redundancy, failure in a test, a bereavement or a diagnosis of ill health). Most life events include both positive and negative aspects – as suggested in Point 4 of the manifesto of the life course perspective – so our feelings may be mixed and complex. Sometimes, the number of events we are experiencing is too few for our needs at the time, and we are bored. If we are lucky, the number is just right, and we are excited, energized and motivated but not snowed under. At other times the number or magnitude of our life events is so great as to leave almost no part of our lives unmolested, and we may feel overwhelmed, out of control, lost and powerless. Our assessments are not fixed, and our evaluation of our situation may vacillate wildly. Nonetheless, as occupational therapists, you will frequently work with people who are experiencing life events that are both very significant and very painful. This chapter sets out to encourage a theoretical understanding of life events that can be applied practically to enable clients to live as fulfilling a life as possible, in the way that they want.

How we react to other people's life events will to some extent depend on whether we, too, have undergone a similar experience, how we dealt with it, what our feelings were about it and what meaning it had for us. To take a simple example, if a close friend suffers a bereavement, perhaps the death of a parent, our response will be influenced by, among other things, whether we have experienced a similar loss, how recent that experience was, how raw it remains and how we dealt with it. Also significant could be whether we received help and support from other people, and the effectiveness of that support. If our friend's experience seems beyond anything we have gone through, we may feel helpless, uncomprehending and fearful of the knowledge that we still have such losses ahead of us. We may feel unsympathetic or even irritated since we do not understand the experience and feelings of our friend. It is worth bearing in mind that we will not have had experience of all the situations that our clients find themselves in, and certainly, since no two events are ever identical, any experience we seem to have shared may give us insight but will never be exactly replicated. For this reason alone, a good grasp of life event theory is important in order to help us make the leap of imagination we need if we are to offer our clients understanding and respect, and make appropriate decisions about intervention.

It is also important to be aware that life events occurring for one individual affect others in their life space, including family, friends, classmates and colleagues. This impact affects others, in part, according to what is going on in their own lives at the time and what life events they are going through. Thus, the impact of Helen's CVA on her son Andrew's life is influenced by, for example, the fact that not only was he away from home when his mother became ill but also that he was considering moving to America, at least temporarily, on graduation. This applies also to occupational therapists and other health and social care professionals. It can be harder to respond creatively and sympathetically to the life events of others if we are in the midst of several life-changing events ourselves. This notion ties in with the concept of fitness to practise and with the essential and legal duty to protect both children and vulnerable adults (Bichard, 2004). It is the responsibility of all practitioners to consider whether issues in their own life may be making it difficult, impossible or inappropriate for them to work with clients. This is one reason why reflection on your own life is a thread running through many of the Learning Tasks in this text. To be maximally effective as practitioners we need insight into our own past and present experience of life events in order that we can unravel our reactions and see more clearly the needs, goals and possible options of the clients we work with. Learning Task 3.1 represented a first stage in this process.

As occupational therapists, you need to do more than identify and understand the significant life events in your own and your clients' lives. You need also to be able to navigate yourself, and help clients navigate their way, through these experiences. A model put forward by Goodman *et al.* (2006) strives both to identify key factors influencing our ability to cope with life events and change and to provide a framework for working with clients to identify and develop their resources for managing them. For reasons that will be instantly obvious, it is known as the '4-S' model.

Coping with life events: the '4-S' model

Goodman *et al.*'s (2006) model is based on consideration of people's responses to a range of positive and negative significant life events. It rests on three main pillars:

1. The key factors that influence a person's ability to cope with major life events can be grouped into four categories:
   a. the *situation* the person is in (i.e. the nature of the life event in question)
   b. the *self* of the person experiencing the life event
   c. the *support* available to the person
   d. the *strategies* for coping that the person has access to.
2. The various factors under each of these headings can either help or hinder the process of coping with a life event or transition, so that each person can be though of as possessing a set of 'assets and liabilities', 'facilitating and inhibiting forces', 'advantages and disadvantages' or 'strengths and weaknesses' in each of the domains of situation, self, support and strategies.
3. The pattern of a person's assets and liabilities can be assessed through a type of cost/benefit analysis, and this can be used as a basis for designing interventions aimed at strengthening the assets and weakening the liabilities, thus enhancing the person's capacity to manage the life event.

The four key domains in the '4-S' model are summarized below. Within each section, you are asked to apply that aspect of the framework to our case study (pp. 6–11), to a personal transition you have experienced and/or to the experience of one of your clients.

Situation

'Situation variables' refer to characteristics of the life event itself. Whilst this is a valuable way of thinking about life events, it is important that, as client-centred practitioners, you remember that the event per se is less important than its meaning for the individual. Thus, the need to use a walking stick after a knee operation may not seem, on the face of it, to require a major adjustment, but for the client who has negative perceptions of using a walking stick – perhaps interpreting it as an indicator that he or she is becoming old and frail – its significance may be enormous.

From the large number of possible variables that could be used to describe life events (Reese & Smyer, 1983), Goodman *et al.* (2006) select eight as particularly likely to have an impact on people's ability to cope: *trigger, timing, controllability, role change, duration, previous experience, concurrent stress* and *assessment*.

- *Trigger:* This concerns how and why the life event occurred. How did it begin? Was it anticipated (for example a marriage) or unanticipated (for example the unexpected discovery of a partner's infidelity), externally triggered (for example a friend dying suddenly) or internally triggered (realizing your health is not going to improve), a clearly identifiable event (moving to a new area) or an intangible non-event (a decline of social networks)? From the case study we can see that Helen's heart attack was unanticipated, internally triggered and clearly identifiable. Not all life events have such a clear-cut beginning. Thus, when Ranjiv met and married Sarah, this may well have set in motion his gradual transition from an Asian to a more Western way of life and sense of identity.

- *Timing:* You may recall from the manifesto of the life course perspective in Chapter 1 that we are working from the belief that the timing of life events within a person's life course is a significant factor in how those events are perceived and handled. Many conditions that bring clients into the care of occupational therapy services are associated with a particular life stage: osteoporosis, arthritis, heart disease or dementia, for example. Coping with such conditions is recognized as a likely developmental task for the later stages of life. When such conditions occur earlier in the life course than is held to be the norm, there is often a sense that this is unfair, and that the events are 'off time'. They will frequently leave the individual feeling out of step with others of their age and generation. Helen, at 52 years of age, might have been the first in her similar-aged social circle to have suffered a heart attack. It certainly came as a shock to Mary, Helen's mother, to realize that heart attacks really could happen to people of her daughter's age. It may never have occurred to her that Helen could suffer a life-threatening illness before she did. It is also quite likely never to have occurred to Richard that his mother could possibly die before he left school. Such events may seem contrary to the natural order of things and contradict our taken-for-granted view of the nature of the life course. This can add to the difficulties of accepting and adjusting to such situations. When working with clients, it is not only their medical condition that you need to consider, but also the practical and emotional impact of its timing within the client's life course.

- *Controllability:* Life events vary considerably in the extent to which their occurrence, progress and/or outcome are under our control, and you will find that clients may overestimate or under-estimate how much they can influence the events that punctuate their life course. Some will spend much energy railing against conditions that cannot be changed, whilst others will fail to exert what influence they can over their situation. The issue here is not only the actual degree of control we have over our life events but also the degree of control we believe or perceive ourselves to have. Whilst this belief may to some extent be a part of our per-sonality – as is proposed in Rotter's (1966, 1990) much studied notion of a relatively stable internal versus external locus of control – it can also vary across situations, and across time in relation to a particular life event. Exploring with clients their understanding of the extent and limits of what they can do to influence their situation is an important part of promoting self-directed and independent living.

It is important to realize also that, whilst the occurrence of a life event may be beyond our control, our response to it may be within our power, at least to some degree. Think, for example, about Brian (Helen's sister and Mary's eldest child). Initially, he tried to take control of the situation, possibly seeing it as his responsibility as the self-appointed 'head of the family'. He dis-covered, however, both that the situation was not totally control-lable and that others (including his sister and mother) could further scupper his attempts to take charge. To his credit, he is adapting to this situation and, whilst still supporting them both, he is allowing Helen and Mary more space to determine their own future.

- *Role change:* As occupational therapists, you will frequently be concerned with helping clients come to terms with life events that trigger the loss of some roles (for example the role of employee or of participant in a range of physically active and demanding sports) and the assumption of others (perhaps patient, or 'disabled person'). Your clients may have very definite views about what is entailed in being ill or dependent, and you need to be aware of what expectations and assumptions they may have of the 'sick role' and of the role of their carers (including occupational therapists). For much of your time, you will also be concerned with helping clients make adaptations to roles that will continue, but in a changed form. New ways may need to be found to carry out the tasks that comprise the activities of daily living, or social participation.

- *Duration:* A life event that triggers a permanent change will be regarded differently from one whose impact is assumed to be temporary. Clearly, for example, a fractured limb is very different from amputation. In particular, negative aspects of a change may be easier to accept if it is known they will be of limited duration. However, the duration of a change may be uncertain, and this can be even more stressful and unsettling. See how Helen's relatives have very different assumptions about the likely rate and extent of her recovery. Furthermore, a change assumed initially to be temporary may turn out to be permanent (or vice versa), demonstrating how the assessment of a life event is a continuing, dynamic process rather than a once-and-for-all judgement.

- *Previous experience:* Generally, we learn from experience, and if we have successfully weathered a particular kind of life event in the past this will give us both the skills and the confidence to do so again in the future. However, if we experienced past life events as overwhelming and our attempts to resolve them as unsatisfactory, this could decrease our perception of our ability to cope with other life events in the future. Even if the balance between our assets and liabilities has shifted and in theory become more favourable, how we perceive our capabilities has a tremendous effect on how we deal with and cope with life events.

- *Concurrent stress:* The amount and nature of stresses elsewhere in clients' lives will influence their experience of, and ability to cope with, any one particular life event. Furthermore, life events frequently do not occur one at a time, but instead come tumbling one on top of the other. A life event in one arena of life may be the trigger for numerous other changes on other fronts. Consider how Helen's heart attack causes Andrew not only to reassess his role and relationship vis-à-vis his mother but also to rethink his entire future, notably whether or not to continue with his plans to spend a couple of years in America. This may, for example, negatively affect the extent to which he is able to cope with the day-to-day stresses of dealing with his mother's illness. It is possible that it may also have an effect on his social relationships – perhaps he has friends, or a girlfriend, who will be affected by the choices he makes. This will inevitably affect how he handles his mother's situation.

- *Assessment:* The nature of a life event, in terms of the person's assessment of its nature, source, timing, controllability, magnitude, duration and familiarity, will contribute to whether the life event is viewed as positive or negative. Because of this, it is risky to make general assumptions about how a particular life event will be assessed. Individual differences are to be expected. Thus, in our case study, Mary, Brian, Katie, Richard, Alison and Sarah are all seeing things from very different and individual standpoints.

Having summarized some of the key situational factors influencing how people experience and cope with significant life events, we suggest that you turn now to Learning Task 3.2 and examine two of your own life events in more detail.

Learning Task 3.2   Situational characteristics of personal life events

In this task, you are asked to explore the nature of significant life events by comparing and contrasting in relation to the eight key situation dimensions discussed in the text *two distinctly different life events* that you have experienced. The events can be positive or negative, recent or not so recent.

First, at the top of a blank page in your Learning Journal, describe in 10–20 words the two life events that you are going to examine.

Now answer the following questions in relation to both events:

- *Trigger:* What set off the event? Was it expected or unexpected? Wanted or unwanted? Externally or internally triggered?
- *Timing:* When in the life course did the event occur? How did the timing of the event affect the way you experienced and managed it?
- *Control:* To what extent did you control the occurrence of the life event? In what ways did you control the way it progressed?
- *Role change:* What changes in role did the life event involve?
- *Duration:* How long did the life event go on for? Did it result in permanent or temporary change in your life space?
- *Previous experience:* Had you experienced similar life events in the past? How did this affect the present life event?
- *Concurrent stress:* What and how great were other stresses and demands you were facing at the time?
- *Assessment:* Did you view the experience as positive or negative? In what ways did your assessment change over time?

Finally, compare and contrast the two life events you have considered. In what ways are they similar? In what ways are they different?

Self

Whereas the 'situation' variable in the '4-S' framework refers to the nature of the life event under consideration, 'self' refers to the person experiencing the event. It refers to their personal and demographic characteristics, and to their psychological characteristics and personality. For each individual, these factors represent a unique network of assets and liabilities. The client-centred focus of occupational therapy and other health and social care professions means that it is the self of your client that is at the heart of the work you do.

Personal and demographic characteristics – where we 'sit' within our society as a consequence of factors such as our age and life stage, socio-economic status, gender, ethnicity and state of health – can give us each access to widely different resources. These resources bear directly on the opportunities and hurdles facing us as we confront major life events, and on how we perceive and assess our life. Do we have sufficient contacts, know-how, financial wherewithal and social power to call upon the resources that are available to help us manage major life events? If we are living on the margins of society, our access to social resources is likely to be limited. Thus, the very old and the very young frequently have limited social and financial power (Pilgrim, 1997), and it may fall to their carers to ensure that their needs are given due attention. This may indeed be a part of your own professional role. Factors such as poverty, social isolation and communication or mobility difficulties can all represent hurdles that can stand in the way of the effective management of life events. In the course of your work, you will often be called upon to help clients overcome or compensate for these difficulties.

As well as our personal and demographic circumstances, we each have psychological resources or characteristics that mediate between the demands placed on us and our response to those demands. Thus, people approach the same life event differently, depending on their level of maturity. Children may not have reached the stage of cognitive maturity where they can analyse life events using abstract thinking. People's location within other frameworks – for example Erikson's (1994) sequence of psychosocial stages and crises – will, similarly, influence the way they experience and respond to life events.

A client's personality is also important. Psychological inventories can measure any number of particular personality traits, but those likely to be of major relevance to occupational therapy professional practice include the often overlapping characteristics of self-esteem, locus of control, flexibility, optimism and hardiness. A thread running through many of these constructs is the extent to which individuals believe themselves to be capable of influencing the course of their life. Again, the issue of controllability – actual or perceived – is crucial.

Turn now to Learning Task 3.3 to consider the 'self' characteristics of a client you have worked with recently, and how this influenced the ways in which they managed their situation.

Learning Task 3.3   How a client's personal resources (or self) can help and hinder

Consider the 'self' characteristics of a client you have worked with recently. In what ways has each of the following operated as an 'asset' and/or as a 'liability'?

- *Personal and demographic characteristics*
  - age and life stage
  - ethnicity
  - socio-economic status
  - state of health
  - gender
- *Psychological characteristics*
  - self-esteem
  - flexibility
  - locus of control
  - hardiness
  - optimism

Please note that this is really a 'both/and' rather than an 'either/or' question because any one characteristic may represent an asset in some respects, or in some situations, and a liability in others.

Think also about the balance or ratio between the client's 'assets' and 'liabilities' in the area of personal resources. In what ways did this ratio change during the time you worked with the client?

A crucial element of self that relates to implementing change is that of motivation, and of particular relevance here is a model of intentional change proposed by Prochaska *et al.* (1992) and developed on the basis of their work with people with alcohol problems. It has had a significant impact on the understanding and practice of health professionals, not least because it suggests what type of intervention may be most appropriate at different points in the cycle of change, thereby enabling practitioners to 'start where their client is'. Prochaska *et al.*'s work usefully demonstrates that if you do not take into account the client's motivation and readiness to change this, then much of your work will have no effect. The model is represented diagrammatically in Figure 3.1, and the different stages are summarized below. Their relevance to you as occupational therapists stems not least from how it suggests you may think about matching interventions to your client's current position in the cycle of intentional change.

1. *Precontemplation:* At this stage a person has no intention of changing a particular behaviour within the foreseeable future; the attitude is 'As far as I'm concerned, I don't have a problem' or 'I suppose I have faults but there's nothing that I really need to change'. Suggesting action programmes to a client at this stage in the cycle is unlikely to be productive; the client is not ready to engage. More helpful would be exploring the client's circum-

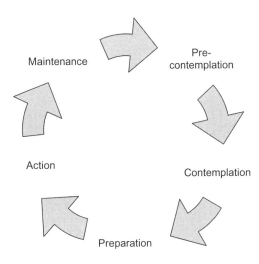

Figure 3.1 The cycle of intentional change (adapted from Prochaska *et al.*, 1992)

stances and discussing some of the areas where change may be beneficial and why.

2. *Contemplation:* At this stage, there is an awareness that a problem exists and the individual is seriously considering doing something about it, but he or she is not yet ready to commit him- or herself to change. Typically, thoughts may be along the lines of 'I have a problem and I really think I should work on it' or 'I've been thinking that I may want to change something about myself'. Here the task is to encourage clients to hasten their walk to a run. Try to build on clients' ideas and suggestions, encouraging them to see the benefits and possibilities of change and the disadvantages of not taking action. It is perfectly possible, of course, that your client will remain unmoved and will choose not to change.

3. *Preparation:* At this stage, there is an immediate intention to change, combined with some small, or so far unsuccessful, steps in the direction of change. This stage has characteristics both of the preceding (that is contemplation) and the subsequent (that is action) stages. The client probably needs assistance with planning and getting started on the action to be taken. The development of clear goals and action plans (discussed in more detail in Chapter 6) can be crucial here. Encouragement and the experience of even some small successes can help to boost the client's sense of confidence in the steps to be taken and a feeling of being able to achieve the goals that have been set.

4. *Action:* Individuals at this stage embody the adages that 'actions speak louder than words' and 'seeing is believing'. They are modifying their behaviour, experiences or environment in order to improve their situation. This can represent a crucial point in the change process: it is where the client is beginning to test out new ways of being and behaving. This is considered further in Chapter 4. At this stage clients tend to feel positive (although possibly still somewhat anxious), higher in mood than previously and more in control. Their self-belief tends to be strong and they may express themselves in phrases such as 'I'm really working hard to change' or 'Anyone can talk about change, but I'm actually doing it'. At this stage clients are largely self-motivated and getting good feedback from successful behaviours. Your role is to offer frequent encouragement and back-up from the sidelines, supporting your clients and helping them to assess their progress and to modify their goals and action plans as necessary.

5. *Maintenance:* During this stage, the gains attained during the action phase are consolidated and people work to prevent relapse. Typical thinking is along the lines of 'I may need a boost right now to help me maintain the changes I've already made' and 'What do I need to do to stop my problem re-emerging?' This is often the trickiest time, especially as it is fairly open-ended. The client has achieved the behavioural change and, with time, any euphoria or sense of achievement at having done something about the issue may pass. Yet there is still work to do to maintain the new behaviour. Hard-won changes may now become boring or seem unimportant, and old behaviours or habits may seem very attractive. Energy and motivation to keep going may falter. It is also at this stage that some supportive stability zones may begin to drop away. Courses of physiotherapy or rehabilitation programmes might have come to an end. Visits and phone calls from family members and friends may lessen as they become distracted by other crises. Alternatively, they may assume that their work is done and so return to other preoccupations. It can be very useful to clients if you are able to maintain some review contact with them in order to provide encouragement and support until the new behaviour is so embedded that it has become habitual.

As many of us know from experience, not all new or desired behaviour is maintained. Lapses may occur, resulting in the cycle of change starting again. Think for a moment of any lapsed New Year resolutions that you have made, perhaps your decision to take up a healthy exercise or eating programme or to give up smoking or spend more wisely. Can you fit your experience into this cycle of intentional change? What or who might have helped you maintain your new behaviour for longer? The following section considers what (or, specifically, who) might have helped you keep on target.

Support

Think about the ideas of the personal life space and of stability zones that were introduced in the previous chapter. Our relationships with other people figure significantly in both of these concepts, a key factor being the support such relationships can provide in helping us implement and manage change. In terms of our capacity to cope with life events, the level and type of support we receive from others can be of crucial importance, and it is generally accepted that there is a positive relationship between social support and health (Langford *et al.*, 1997). It is generally our informal network – our friends, family, neighbours, colleagues and other associates – that we turn to first when we find ourselves faced with crises, challenges or uncertainties. It behoves occupational therapists and other health or social care professionals to remember that they are frequently the final rather than the first port of call, and to involve and harness clients' personal networks and resources to support them as they cope with the consequences of the events that have brought them into your orbit. Helen is fortunate in having many people concerned for her welfare, and helping those people translate their concern into productive support could greatly assist Helen in her recovery and rehabilitation.

In terms of the kind of support that could be provided by a client's social circle, Kahn (1979) distinguishes between the functions of affect, affirmation and aid. *Affective* transactions are those that involve expressions of liking, admiration, respect or love. Transactions involving *affirmation* confirm the appropriateness or rightness of some action or statement, whilst transactions expressing *aid* may offer any number of practical, material and cognitive forms of assistance, including things, money, time, advice, guidance and entitlements.

It is also important to remember that not all social relations are constructive. By their mere existence, social networks have a social-integration effect (Antonucci & Depner, 1982), giving us a niche in society with norms, expectations and obligations. We may appreciate this as a source of security, or instead spurn it as an unwelcome and unpalatable restriction. Most commonly, perhaps, we feel a bit of both, depending on our current circumstances. Family networks, for example, can be a source of both great succour and great stress. Furthermore, on entering a network we may welcome some linkages, but not others. At work and within our family we may experience some relationships that are constructive and supportive, and others that are counterproductive. Members of our personal networks may, intentionally or otherwise, reinforce dysfunctional behaviours, restrict the resources we may potentially call upon or in other ways undermine our efforts to change (Mechanic, 1999). How helpful would it be, for example, to restrict acceptance of support to members of the family, as Mary in our case study would like?

It may also be the case that the support offered is inappropriate, offering advice, perhaps, when emotional support is needed. People in your client's family or social network may assume that what worked for them will also be the best route forward for your client. There may be times when in your work with clients you have to negotiate your way through complex and contradictory support networks in order to secure and facilitate that which is best for the person you are working with.

Thus, both the sustaining and destructive potential of social networks must be recognized. Passing through life events is likely to have an impact – for better, for worse or for both – on people's interpersonal relations. On the one hand, support networks may be mobilized in response to some life events, as when friends rally round to support Helen and her family. On the other hand, established networks may be disrupted. If, for instance, Helen is no longer able to attend the meetings of the local horticultural society, she may lose the support offered, perhaps implicitly rather than explicitly, by her fellow enthusiasts.

In this section, several references have been made to the support available to Helen and her family. Learning Task 3.4 invites you to think about this more systematically.

Learning Task 3.4   Social support networks

Look back at the genogram you constructed for the Case family. Think, in particular, about who in the family has offered support to Helen during her experience of a CVA and its aftermath.

- Make a list of *who* you think has supported Helen.
- What *type* of support did they provide? Think about the extent to which they were each able or potentially able to:
  - make Helen feel liked or loved
  - make Helen feel respected or admired
  - be someone that Helen could confide in
  - support or agree with Helen's thoughts and actions
  - provide immediate, short-term assistance
  - provide regular, consistent assistance over a long period.
- Are there examples where the support was (or may prove to be) a *liability* rather than or as well as an *asset*?

What about support from occupational therapists or other health and social care professionals? What could their role be?

Think about some of the other people in our case study, Andrew, Richard, Sarah, Chris and Mary, for instance. What support needs may they have at this time? What evidence is there that these needs are being met?

This task is based on the *Norbeck Social Support Questionnaire* (Norbeck *et al.*, 1981, 1983; Gigliotti, 2002). Copies of the questionnaire, along with scoring instructions, details of its background and psychometric properties can be downloaded from http://nurseweb.ucsf.edu/www/ffnorb.htm.

Strategies

Whether we are aware of it or not, we all cope with life events. When we say we cannot cope, what we mean is that we believe our coping is not effective, or that all ways forward seem bleak and unmanageable. Perhaps our coping strategies have not worked. Perhaps we do not know what strategies to employ. Perhaps we do not possess the skills or resources we believe to be necessary, or we are not confident about the outcomes. In the face of life exigencies, we could employ any number of specific responses, some more effective and appropriate than others. Think about the many different coping strategies adopted by the members of Helen's family in response to her illness. We all have a range of coping strategies that we bring to bear on life event experiences. Use Learning Task 3.5 to consider what some of these strategies may be.

Learning Task 3.5   What are your coping strategies?

This time, the Learning Task asks you to reflect on and analyse your own experience.

Identify a significant challenge you have faced recently and pair up with a friend or colleague, taking turns to interview each other about how you each coped with this significant event in your life:

- What strategies did you use?
- Which were the most effective strategies, and why?
- How might you handle a similar situation differently if it arose again?

Discuss with your partner how the knowledge/understandings you have just gained may be useful in your work with clients.

It is almost inevitable that a person's repertoire of coping strategies can be expanded and/or used more effectively, and this is a topic considered further in Chapter 5. Whereas the 'self' variable refers to what individuals bring to life events by virtue of who they are, and the 'support' variable relates to the interpersonal resources they have available to them, 'strategies' refers to what people actually do. Generally speaking, it is easier to change what we do rather than who we are.

Facilitating clients' development of new strategies or skills is a key role for all health and social care professionals. Of course, this, in turn, can lead to changes in the way clients see themselves, in their personal resources and in their social circumstances. In other words, the development of additional strategies for coping with change can promote the strengthening of self and the enhancement of support. Small beginnings in one area can lead to large developments across the board. The four 'S' categories should not be seen as totally independent; indeed, one category may well have a profound and significant effect upon another.

Many of the key strategies that you use in your professional work with clients as they address areas of change in their life space can be seen as contributing to clients' management of transitions, their coping with stress and their management of problem areas within their life. These generic developmental tasks form the focus of the next three chapters.

4. *Transition and Loss*

Life events are more than milestones on a map which chart our journey from cradle to grave. They are also processes over time that can change us in significant ways and alter both the nature of our current life space and the direction of our future life course. You will find that the experience of many of your clients will have forced them into profound, often involuntary, and possibly sudden reassessments of their self-image, their sense of who they are. Thus, Helen Case's experience has required her to move from seeing herself as a healthy, physically active, independent person to seeing herself as a sick hospital patient with, possibly, long-term health difficulties. This requires a major process of psychological identity transformation that involves adjusting to a changed body and to changed functional abilities. It is life events such as these, events which can be thought of as personal transitions or turning points, that are the focus of this chapter.

A transition can be said to occur when 'an event or non-event results in a change in assumptions about oneself and the world and thus requires a corresponding change in one's behaviour and relationships' (Schlossberg, 1981, p. 5). This is only one of several possible definitions and, indeed, the area represents a definitional quagmire. The notion of life change is crucial, but, beyond that, there are many definitions emphasizing different features (Ruble & Seidman, 1996). Some definitions emphasize a change in status (for example from single to married, from student to practitioner); others, the magnitude of the change or its consequences. For our purposes, and in keeping with the client-centred emphasis of this book and occupational therapy practice, a more subjective rather than objective definition is appropriate, hence the value of Schlossberg's definition, which prioritizes changes in the person's self-definition rather than his or her behaviour or social status.

Wethington *et al.*'s (1997) definition of what they term a 'turning point' rather than a transition is valuable as a more comprehensive checklist of significant characteristics.

A turning point:

- is a period or point in time when a person undergoes a major transformation in views about the self, commitments to important relationships or involvement in significant life roles
- involves a fundamental shift in the meaning, purpose or direction of a person's life
- includes a self-reflective awareness of, or insight into, the significance of the change
- can be brought on by major life events, chronic difficulties, normative life transitions, minor events and internal, subjective changes (such as self-insights or re-interpretations of past experiences)
- can be positive or negative in character.

Perhaps you have already started to relate these concepts of transition and turning points to your own experience or to that of clients you have worked with. Learning Task 4.1 invites you to do this systematically.

Learning Task 4.1   Identifying transitions and turning points

- Generate a list of experiences you have encountered that meet the criteria of transitions and turning points. It may be that the life events you listed in Learning Task 3.1 (p. 54) and considered in Learning Task 3.2 (p. 61) will fit the bill. Try, however, not to restrict yourself to these examples.
- Now think of clients you have worked with, and identify transitions and turning points they were facing at the time.
- Think about what marked these experiences out as transitions or turning point, and then, if possible, compare notes with a partner or small group of colleagues.
- Keep a record of these examples in your Learning Journal and keep them in mind as you read through the rest of this chapter. Consider the extent to which you can recognize the stages of transition in both your own and your clients' experiences. The next Learning Task will ask you explicitly to plot your own transition through these different stages in relation to two different experiences.

We do not yet know whether Helen's CVA will mark a turning point in her life, but the likelihood is that it will. If it means that her mother will no longer be able to live with her, then it might trigger a turning point in her mother's life as well. If her elder son feels that, on finishing university, he must find work near his home rather than take a planned job in North America, it will mark a turning point in his life also. The ripples from a major event in the life of one person can travel a very long way and set up equally major life events for others, which in their turn ripple onwards and affect yet another set of people.

Life events as processes: the dynamics of personal transitions

Terminal illness and bereavement are amongst the most profound of human experiences, and both are often accompanied by not dissimilar emotional and cognitive responses. Thus, Elisabeth Kubler-Ross's (1997) work on death and dying has provided one of the most influential and widely disseminated models of transition. It is a landmark example of a life event being viewed as a long-term process rather than as a point-in-time occurrence. The model proposes five distinct, but overlapping, stages in the process of facing and coming to terms with death. The stages are not necessarily progressive in that not everyone will proceed through them all. Whilst they are not exactly comparable, the sequence is similar to John Bowlby's (1980) phases of brief grief, and both are summarized in Table 4.1.

These formulations have had an immense impact on the attitude and practice of professionals working with the dying and the bereaved, but they have been criticized as suggesting too prescriptively that there is a right and, therefore, by implication, a wrong way of experiencing loss. It is, indeed, crucial to be aware that each person's experience of transition is unique. We should never say 'I know exactly how you feel' to another person, for we cannot ever fully know how they feel. However, this does not mean that each transitional experience is completely unique and has no features in common with any other experience. Indeed, there is considerable evidence to suggest (Hopson & Adams, 1976; Hopson & Scally, 1997) that, irrespective of the nature of the transition, there is a general pattern of reaction to significant life events, albeit a pattern with a myriad of variations. Being aware of this reaction can help

Table 4.1 Stages of dying and grief.

Kubler-Ross's stages of dying	Bowlby's stages of grief
Denial: the refusal to believe a terminal diagnosis	**Shock:** a sense of numbness and urge to deny the truth of the loss
Anger: often directed at family members or medical staff	**Pining:** a stage of yearning, anger and protest
Bargaining: negotiating with God or some other higher being for more time	
Depression: beginning to acknowledge and mourn the impending loss	**Disorganization and despair:** characterized by feelings of depression
Acceptance: acquiescing to and no longer fighting the inevitable	**Readjustment:** involving some sort of reconciliation to or acceptance of the new situation

you as you work with your clients to develop programmes of care with them that are attuned to their current location in this roller-coaster of thoughts and feelings. Recognizing that the sequence described in the transition cycle is 'normal' (that is not inherently pathological) and 'normative' (that is experienced by others as well as our self) can provide hope, a sense of direction and reassurance that things need not always remain the same, that just as others have experienced tragedy and lived through it to face the future so may we.

Despite wide individual differences in the timing and intensity of each stage, most of us can recognize the following sequence of reaction in our response to major upheavals in our life space resulting from significant life events:

1. Shock or immobilization

The initial response to a major life event or to important news suggesting major upheaval to the life space is frequently one of shock. This applies whether the event comes completely out of the blue (as with Helen's CVA) or was at some level half expected (for example the diagnosis of an illness). Even long-anticipated life events can leave us confused and bewildered when they eventually occur.

There are many metaphorical phrases that sum up this stage: being 'frozen in our tracks', being 'knocked sideways' and being 'stunned into silence'. We can see how Helen's son Andrew responded in this way when he first learnt of his mother's illness. It is not unusual for the sense of mental and emotional numbing to be mirrored physically: people may feel cold, move and speak slowly or feel very tired.

A key feature of this stage is that our powers of comprehension and reasoning will desert us. For a greater or lesser time, depending on the degree of shock that we experience, we will not be able to take in much of what is said to us. It will 'all go over our head', to use another metaphor. We will not be in a good frame of mind to make major decisions. It is important to think about this in relation to work with clients; it is often necessary to give clients several opportunities to take in information, for example, or for them to have another person there with them who can check and assist their understanding at a later date.

2. Reaction and minimization

The boundaries between the different phases of the transition cycle are rarely clear cut, and so it tends to be only gradually that the emotional paralysis of the shock phase fades, to be replaced by a reaction in the form of a sharp mood swing. This swing of mood may, even for undesirable events, move in a positive direction – for example, 'Well, at least I know what's wrong with me now; that's better than the uncertainty' – but more often, clients' mood levels will drop, to anything from mild disappointment to deep despair.

After this initial reaction, there is frequently a stage during which clients seek to deny the extent of their problem or minimize the extent of its likely impact. A positive reaction to a negative life event can itself be seen as a form of minimization or suppression of the trauma that helps the person avoid or escape from confronting its full impact. Similarly, attempts by clients to 'put a brave face on things' and search for positive or optimistic interpretations of the situation can help them escape the disorientation of the shock stage and the distress of the reaction phase.

Many other clichés capture the essence of this phase. 'Well, it could have been worse,' a client may say. They may put the whole issue 'to the back of their mind' and may resist the efforts of others to make them face up to what has happened. Alternatively, they may confront the trauma with the stereotypical 'stiff upper lip', reflecting cultural taboos about expressing emotions in public, or to people outside the family. This was the stance of Helen Case's mother, Mary, and doubtless reflects the values and practice of her background and generation as well as of her individual views and personality traits. She exerted pressure on members of the immediate family to strive to meet all of her daughter's current and future needs – not admitting to the possibility that this may be impossible, unrealistic and not necessarily in Helen's best interests.

A risk is that this minimization is interpreted by others as reconciliation to the life event. The person may seem to have got over it with admirable ease and speed (possibly to the relief of family, friends and professionals, all of whom may be uncomfortable and/or distressed about the situation and may find the other person's distress difficult to deal with). However, whilst minimization can be valuable in giving a person a breathing space during which to 'regain their bearings', in the longer term it gets in the way of open and creative decision-making. Minimization distorts the reality of the situation and, therefore, can inhibit movement through later stages of the transition cycle. It is, however, very common, and it is important that health and social care professionals recognize this and do not assume that the client no longer needs help.

3. Self-doubt

With time, it becomes harder to ignore or minimize the consequences and implications of significant life events. As the reality of the change becomes inescapable, self-doubt often creeps in, frequently grounded in a sense of personal powerlessness and/or guilt. This can lead to feelings of depression, possibly with periods of sadness and apathy being interspersed with bouts of anger and anxiety. The person's mood is on a downward slide during this phase, and represents a time when mental health is especially vulnerable. This is the position that Helen is now in. The immediate physical crisis is passed, and this lull after the storm means Helen can no longer avoid facing up to what has happened to her, and its possible long-term consequences. Her continuing physical and cognitive difficulties have undermined her confidence in her health and in her capacity to cope. Whilst heart attacks are far from unknown in women in their early fifties, they are not the norm; and Helen's sense that her experience is 'off time' is likely to add to her difficulties in coming to terms with it.

Unfortunately, by this stage support from other people might have lessened, partly because the person is thought to have recovered from the event, or at least reconciled themselves to the new situation. If Helen's physical and medical needs are being attended to, the people around her might be less aware of her emotional and support needs. It is also the case that people are often unaware of how much time is needed to come to terms with a major loss, and a slide into sadness at this stage may be seen as wallowing in self-pity, self-indulgent and blameworthy. It is very important for those working with a client going through a major transition to recognize each stage for what it is, so that interventions can be timely and appropriate. At this stage what is needed is acceptance and acknowledgement of the client's feelings, and recognition of their right to feel as they do.

4. Accepting reality and letting go

Throughout the previous stages, the person's world view has been grounded in 'life as it was' prior to the experience that triggered the transition. During this fourth stage, however, attention is directed away from the past and focused on the future, thereby loosening the hold of the past and clearing the way for the person to face the realities of the present and the challenges of the future. This is the point at which interventions that work towards making changes and moving on can start to become appropriate. It is important to bear in mind, however, that clients are likely to move back and forth between stages, and that the non-judgemental acceptance and support which was so crucial in the early stages of the transition remains important throughout. For many people, periods of optimism and forward planning will alternate with periods of apathy, regret and sadness.

Occupational therapists can have a particularly important and prominent role during this and the next stage in the transition cycle. The practical activities, skills and support that are major tools of the occupational therapist's trade in working with clients are grounded in what the clients can do in the present. This, by focusing on the here and now, allows the person to move away from the past. It helps clients look forward to the future rather than backwards to a past to which they can never return. By focusing on successful achievement in the present, occupational therapists and other health and social care professionals can help clients begin to develop a sense of control and efficacy that contrasts with previously felt powerlessness and lack of self-worth.

However, it is important – to use another metaphor – not to throw the baby out with the bathwater. When we 'let go', we do not normally 'put the past behind us' and leave it there. More usually, ties are loosened and renegotiated, rather than broken completely (Klass *et al.*, 1996). Links with the past need not and, indeed, should not be totally severed. Remember how, in Chapter 2, we considered the notion of stability zones – anchors that sustain us and hold us steady when the rest of our world is in turmoil? The 'belongings' that we identify as stability zones are frequently objects that link us to our past. They may include mementoes of people who are no longer physically present in our life but who remain important to us, and whose memory and influence we want to preserve. We may call on these people in our imagination and wonder what they would have suggested that we do in a particular situation, we may speculate about how they would have felt about various decisions that we make, and what they would have made of our triumphs and our disasters. But, at the same time, we do have to come to terms with the reality that they are no longer around in the way that they were in the past.

So, letting go does not involve a total severance from the past, for our past is a large part of what makes us who we are today. Rather, the past needs to be integrated into a coherent and durable personal life story. Thus, Worden (1995), writing specifically about bereavement, identifies four tasks of mourning: to accept the reality of the loss, to work through the pain of grief, to adjust to an environment in which the deceased is missing, and to emotionally relocate the deceased and move on with life. The fourth task was amended from an earlier version (1983), where it was identified as the withdrawal of emotional energy from the deceased and its reinvestment in another relationship. The new formulation represents a far more explicit valuing of the person's past and of its continuing influence in the present. The same applies to other aspects of a person's past. Someone who sustains a serious back injury whilst playing rugby and now needs a wheelchair to get about may, at least initially, want nothing further to do with the sport. In time, however, they may be able to carve other meaningful roles for themselves, perhaps in coaching or as a spectator, that both draw on their skills and knowledge and sustain their identity as a keen sports enthusiast.

Nonetheless, letting go and facing the future inevitably involves something of 'a leap in the dark'. Levinson (1990) describes the experience of being in this space between life structures as like being 'adrift on a raft': the land one has left is lost from view, and the new land has not yet appeared on the horizon. Launching oneself into this void can be frightening, leaving us feeling 'all at sea'. Clients may be tempted to rush through this void, and, in so doing, make quick and ill-considered decisions about their future. However, this void is also a time that is rich with possibilities. Bridges (2004) describes it evocatively as a time of 'fertile emptiness'. It may hold options and opportunities of which clients are unaware. It is important for professionals to support clients as they deal with the uncertainty and disorientation of this phase, and encourage them to cast their net widely when thinking about the future. They need also to think creatively in order to maximize the range of possibilities considered by their clients. As a way of helping clients to liberate themselves from imagined as well as real restrictions, it can be valuable to encourage clients to think first of their wildest dreams and ambitions without concern for their feasibility, and only then work backwards to what may be achievable within the immediate future. Are there things that Helen has always wanted to do, but has never had the opportunity? She still may not be able to fulfil these dreams, but putting them into words may sow the seeds of other, more realistic, goals and aspirations.

5. Testing

As with the process of experiential learning that was discussed in Chapter 0, moving through a transition involves activity as well as reflection, and the fifth stage, testing, is a phase where the emphasis on purposeful activity and trying out new situations and ways of doing things is especially pertinent. It is an experimental period during which new activities, lifestyles and ways of coping are tried. It is likely that clients will experience setbacks and disappointments: not all new endeavours will be successful. This is where remaining open to new possibilities and having a range of contingency plans can bear fruit. As an occupational therapist, you can support clients through setbacks, and help them amend or revise plans and goals as they discover both what they want and what it is feasible for them to strive for.

Rapid mood changes may occur as plans are considered and discarded, and as hopes are raised and dashed. Nonetheless, the low point of the transition is past and, taken overall, the person's mood, morale or level of self-esteem is on the rise. Although this process will not necessarily run smoothly, and clients may find that the self-doubt of stage 3 returns on occasions to haunt them, generally the direction of movement is forward, and the 'testings' prove purposeful and rewarding.

6. Search for meaning

After the emotional turmoil of the previous two stages, this sixth phase in the transition cycle is characterized by a conscious striving to make sense of and learn from the experience. It is a healthy form of reflective thinking that can help us appreciate what we have achieved in terms of both outcomes and new skills. It facilitates reconciliation with, and understanding of, the meaning of the change. It is an acknowledgement and celebration of what has been survived, and should not be interpreted as 'morbid dwelling on the past'. Creative therapies involving such things as art, drama, creative writing and storytelling may be useful in helping clients to explore, reflect on, validate and make sense of their experiences.

7. Integration

At this final stage in the transition sequence, whilst there may, as discussed in Chapter 3, be issues around the maintenance of some of the changes the client has instigated (Prochaska *et al.*, 1992), clients can frequently achieve a degree of closure with regard to the event in that it becomes an integral part of how they see themselves. The experience has become a part of who they are, rather than something that happened 'to' them. By this stage, the work of the health and social care professionals will very largely be done, and clients will be living their lives as independently as possible.

However, not all clients will reach this stage of acceptance and equanimity. Some people get stuck at a particular stage or continually go back and forth between stages, never reaching the final point in the cycle. The cycle of responses outlined in this chapter represents a sketch – a probability or a possibility. It is certainly not a straitjacket into which clients and/or their experience should be squeezed. The intensity of the different stages, and the time needed to work through them, varies enormously. Client-centred practice demands that the individual's unique experience takes precedence over any search to categorize the person within any one particular stage of the transition cycle. A valuable way of recognizing this can be to develop an appreciation of your own experience of transition, as implied in Learning Task 4.1. The next activity, Learning Task 4.2, builds on the final bullet point of Learning Task 4.1 by asking you to record systematically your passage through two contrasting transitions.

Learning Task 4.2   Transition analysis

- Using the stages of transition listed below and discussed in the text, plot your own progress through two transitions. Choose one *planned* and one *unplanned* experience.
- To what extent are you able to identify these different stages in your own experience?
  - ○ immobilization
  - ○ reaction: mood swing followed by minimization
  - ○ self-doubt
  - ○ accepting reality and letting go
  - ○ testing
  - ○ searching for meaning
  - ○ integration
- What were the differences in your experience at the time?
- How do you perceive the outcome/experience now?
- Focusing on one of these transitions, consider the impact it might have had, and is possibly still having, on transitions being experienced by members of your family or other significant people in your life space.

The experience of loss

Even transitions that are welcomed and freely chosen involve loss. This, you will recall, is one of the tenets of the life course manifesto, that all change involves both gain and loss (although the balance between them can, of course, vary enormously). We are held by emotional bonds to our current life space, and these bonds, whether we like it or not, resist severance (Parkes, 1971, 1993). This notion underpins the common lament that we 'don't know what we've got until it's gone'. 'Home cooking', 'the family cat', 'the view from the spare bedroom' and 'the tick of the hall clock', for example, are all things that students have told us they experienced as losses when they moved away from their childhood home to go to university, despite being pleased to have moved on, and happy in their new environment. They had been unaware of how important these things had been to them and how, as stability zones, they had operated as oases of security.

Post-traumatic growth

By the same token, gains may emerge even from very challenging life circumstances or changes that seem saturated with loss. A woman abandoned by her husband and with no means of supporting herself may, once she has trained in a new line of work and become financially independent, feel that she has fulfilled potentials she never realized she had. Such experience is known as 'post-traumatic growth' (Tedeschi & Calhoun, 2004; Calhoun & Tedeschi, 2006). Even losses that will always be regretted may lead to some gains. The person incapacitated by illness or made redundant from a job they loved may, nonetheless, fill the gap created in their life space with new and meaningful activities and goals. As an occupational therapist, you can frequently be instrumental in facilitating such positive psychological and behavioural change.

The notion that suffering and distress can trigger positive change is not new; it underpins the 'no pain, no gain' slogan, for example. Growth does not, however, occur as a direct result of the trauma. It is the individual's struggle with the new reality which follows the trauma that is crucial to determining whether and to what extent post-traumatic growth occurs. Whilst the trauma itself may remain a distressing event, those who demonstrate post-traumatic growth are able to find something of value in what happens to them in the aftermath of trauma, in their efforts to cope or survive. Helping clients to face, adapt to, learn from and transcend losses is an important, challenging and frequently rewarding part of your role. Reflecting on the balance between gains and losses in relation to some of your own life experiences is the focus of Learning Task 4.3.

Learning Task 4.3   Gains and losses

- List some of the *positive* changes you have experienced in your life. Note down what it was that made them positive.
  - ○ What was it that you *gained*?
  - ○ Now think about what you *lost* in the process.
- Now list some of the *negative* or *unwanted* changes you have experienced.
  - ○ What did you *lose* in the course of these events?
  - ○ Can you think of anything that you *gained* as a result of these experiences?
  - ○ When did you become aware of any gains – was it at the time or only in retrospect?
  - ○ In what ways has awareness of these gains affected your assessment of the events?

Parkes (1993) visually represents the loss–gain balance in different life changes by using the simple rectangle depicted below. A transition at point 1 represents a life change characterized by overwhelming loss, whilst one at point 8 is experienced as a virtually unequivocal gain.

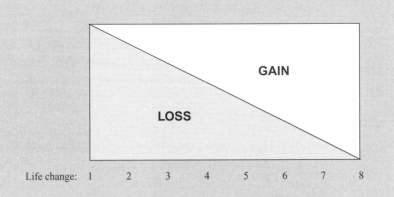

Life change: 1   2   3   4   5   6   7   8

Gain and loss components of life changes (Parkes, 1993)
(Reproduced by permission of Cambridge University Press, from Parkes, C.M. (1993). Bereavement as a psychosocial transition: processes of adaptation to change. In M. S. Stroebe, W. Stroebe & R. Hansson (eds), *Handbook of Bereavement: Theory, Research and Intervention*.)

> - Try to identify life events or transitions with which you are familiar that represent the different ratios of gain to loss at different points on the scale 1–8. Where on this scale would you place some of the transitions you have experienced in your own life? Look back to the case study and note down the gains and losses that we know the following characters have experienced:
>   - Paul
>   - Richard
>   - Sarah
>   - Helen
>   - Brian
>
> What counterbalancing losses and gains did, or might, these events also have triggered? Where would you place these life changes on the loss–gain scale above?

Tedeschi and Calhoun (2004) identify five domains in which post-traumatic growth may be evident. Read through the list and see to what extent you can identify these themes in your answers to Learning Task 4.3:

- An increased appreciation for life in general, and a changed set of priorities that leads to a greater valuing of 'little things' which might previously have gone unnoticed.
- The development of closer, deeper and more meaningful relationships with valued others, along with, possibly, the withdrawal of involvement in less significant relationships. There may be a determination not to waste time on unimportant or uncongenial pursuits.
- An increased recognition of personal strengths, perhaps combined, somewhat paradoxically, with a sense of personal vulnerability. In other words, along with the recognition that bad things can and do happen, there is a sense that 'If I handled that, I can handle more or less anything'.
- The identification of new possibilities and positive life paths that might not otherwise have been considered.
- An increased spiritual and existential appreciation, possibly, but not necessarily, religious. There may be a greater engagement

with fundamental existential questions that is in itself experienced as growth.

In terms of personal factors that may be associated with the development of post-traumatic growth, Tedeschi and Calhoun (2004) conclude:

> Certain kinds of personal qualities – extraversion, openness to experience, and perhaps optimism – may make growth a bit more likely. Initially, the individual typically must engage in coping responses needed to manage overwhelming emotions, but intense cognitive processing of the difficult circumstances also occurs. The degree to which the person is engaged cognitively by the crisis appears to be a central element in this process of posttraumatic growth. The individual's social system may also play an important role in the general process of growth, particularly through the provision of new schemas related to growth, and the empathic acceptance of disclosures about the traumatic event and about growth-related themes. Posttraumatic growth seems closely connected to the development of general wisdom about life, and the development and modification of the individual's life narrative. Although posttraumatic growth has been found to be correlated with a reduction of distress, our thinking is some degree of psychological upset or distress is necessary not only to set the process of growth in motion, but also some enduring upset may accompany the enhancement and maintenance of posttraumatic growth. (pp. 12–13)

Think about clients you have worked with, and note in your Learning Journal instances where they possessed some or all of these qualities. To what extent did they also appear to experience growth in the aftermath of their traumatic experience? How can, or did, occupational therapy interventions promote this?

A 'health warning' about post-traumatic growth

The concept of post-traumatic growth can help occupational therapists in their crucially important task of assisting clients to develop and maintain a sense of hope, even if that hope cannot be for a full return to health or even for a lifespan that extends far into the future. However, it should not be seen as a panacea for all. To assume that post-traumatic growth is a possibility may be to deny the reality of clients' suffering in the present. It is vital that occupational therapists proceed with caution (Tedeschi & Calhoun, 1995, 2004).

It should never be forgotten that post-traumatic growth occurs in the context of suffering and significant psychological struggle, and a focus on growth should not come at the expense of sympathy for the pain and suffering of trauma survivors. For most trauma survivors, growth emerges from the struggle with coping, not from the trauma itself. Post-traumatic growth will, therefore, coexist with distress. Whilst at least to some extent inevitable, life crises, loss and trauma should not be viewed as inherently desirable. It is possible for individuals to mature and develop in meaningful ways without experiencing tragedy or trauma.

All health and social care practitioners should, therefore, first address high levels of emotional distress in their clients, providing the support that can help to make this distress manageable. Allowing time for a distressed client to regain the ability to function cognitively in the aftermath of the trauma will promote the possibility for post-traumatic growth. Active listening – without necessarily trying to offer solutions – can give clients the space to process trauma into growth. As an occupational therapist, it is important that you learn to become comfortable and willing to work with clients as they process existential or spiritual concerns triggered by their trauma. Matters related to growth are best addressed after the individual has had sufficient opportunity to adapt to the aftermath of the trauma. It links most closely to stage 6 in the transition cycle – the search for meaning.

Loss in a life course context

A life course perspective sees not only individual transitions but also whole life stages, as a balance between losses and gains. All life stages, not only those of the so-called 'formative years' involve gains. Thus, whilst many middle-aged parents may be a little sad to see their children move away from the family home into independent adulthood, they may also relish the freedom this affords them to develop new interests or revive old skills that have fallen into abeyance during the demands of the active parenting years.

Similarly, it is not only the stages of later life that involve the experience of loss. The formal attainment of adulthood at age 18 is generally seen as a reason for celebration and congratulation, with scant attention given as to what is being lost. Young people may be bemused and possibly a little embarrassed by their fears for the future and their anxieties about what they are leaving behind (Apter, 2001). We often do not recognize that there are losses as well as gains, even when we move onward and upward in life. Look now at Learning Tasks 4.4, which asks you to consider more systematically this balance between gain and loss at each life stage.

Learning Task 4.4   The gains and losses of different life stages

- Look back at Learning Task 1.4 (Developmental tasks across the life course, p. 23) and at Table 1.1 (Developmental tasks and health issues by life stage, pp. 27–9) and think again about the different stages of life. This time, have in mind the relative balance between loss and gain in the developmental tasks characterizing each stage.
- Select two developmental tasks for each life stage and note down and/or discuss with a partner the ways in which each task may incorporate both gain and loss.
- Consider the relevance to losses other than bereavement of using Worden's (1995) tasks of mourning, which were mentioned earlier. Namely:
  - to accept the reality of the loss
  - to work through the pain of grief
  - to adjust to an environment in which that which has been lost is missing
  - to emotionally relocate that which has been lost and move on with life.

Some gains and losses associated with a particular life stage are normative, and are the consequence of addressing age-associated developmental tasks. Others are non-normative and reflect the individual ups and downs of our particular life course. Alison's loss of her baby when she was in her mid-teens is a case in point. We cannot know whether this will make it harder or easier for her to cope with the life-threatening nature of Helen's illness, but it will almost certainly have an impact one way or another (even though it was something that occurred nearly 30 years ago).

The majority of us will find coping with transitions and significant life events a personal challenge. Indeed, we are likely to experience many of them as stressful. The transitions and life events that your clients are experiencing during the time you are working with them will almost inevitably be accompanied by a degree of stress. Understanding and managing this stress is an important developmental task at all life stages, and is the focus of our next chapter.

5. *Stress and its Management*

Life events, transitions and loss – in other words the topics considered in our previous two chapters – may be saturated with stress. Indeed, it is a truism to say that stress is a scourge of our times. However, whilst modern life can be very stressful, it is debatable whether the stress experienced is at a greater level than, or just differs in source and nature from, that of earlier centuries. Perhaps it is simply that most of us in the developed world have to spend less energy striving to fulfil our basic survival needs for food, shelter, warmth and safety. However, we seem to have put that competitive energy into striving for less concrete goals, which are equally inclined to cause stress, and certainly whilst life may not be so hard for most of us now, it is very much faster, and the pace of change – always a stressor as we have seen in previous chapters – has never been so rapid or so relentless (Sennet, 2006). In line with this, when working through the material in Chapter 3 concerning the significant characteristics of life events, 'concurrent stress' was identified as a factor influencing our capacity to cope with change.

Although it is a tenet of our manifesto of the life course perspective that all life events present opportunities for growth and, indeed, the notion of post-traumatic growth was considered in the previous chapter, it is important not to be too 'Pollyanna-ish' about this. The silver linings in some clouds may be very hard to find. Although, as has been emphasized throughout this work book, we may recognize that the individual's interpretation of an event is likely to be a significant, perhaps the most significant, factor in determining the amount of stress experienced, it is nonetheless possible to make some generalizations about the more objective dimensions of life events and transitions associated with increased levels of stress.

Thus, a higher rather than a lower level of stress is generally associated with experiences that are, as Hopson (1981) suggests, involuntary, unfamiliar, of high magnitude, of high intensity and with an unpredictable or uncertain outcome. Thus, in general, it is involuntary transitions – ones we did not choose and would not have wished to experience – that are the more stressful. We may see them involving loss rather than gain, and they may be forced on us against our will, thereby diminishing our sense of personal control. Stress is also heightened in transitions that are unfamiliar. Our past experience, we may rightly suspect, has not provided us with the opportunity to develop skills with which to cope with the situation in which we now find ourselves. We do not know what is going to be asked of us, or whether we will be able to cope. This being so, the outcome of the transition is more unpredictable (an already mentioned characteristic of stressful transitions). Many of us do not cope easily with uncertainty. Thus, in our case study (pp. 6–11), Brian may find it more stressful to deal with the uncertainty of Helen's recovery than knowing the prognosis is poor. Many of you will have seen the relief felt by clients when they received a clear diagnosis of their condition. In such cases, there is a situation (albeit an undesirable one) to respond to. We have a better sense of what we are dealing with. By contrast, uncertainty is ephemeral, elusive and disconcerting.

Transitions of high magnitude, that is those having an impact on large areas of our life space, are also particularly stressful. It is certainly the case that Helen's experience of a CVA falls into this category. In such instances, more of our stability zones are likely to be disrupted. Transitions of high intensity – those requiring an immediate or at least very rapid response – also place particular strain on us. If they were also unexpected, then you will appreciate, following our discussion of transitions, that the person might be in a state of shock and, therefore, particularly ill-equipped to respond in a rational and thoughtful manner. As an occupational therapist, you will need to take all these factors into account when working with clients.

Of course, many events will have all of the characteristics identified by Hopson (1981) as associated with the heightened experience of stress, Helen's CVA being a case in point. Another key dimension, the unexpectedness of the event, can be a double-edged sword. On the one hand, the opportunity to prepare ourselves emotionally and practically is denied to us when an event occurs suddenly out of the blue, and our sense of shock is likely to be all the greater. On the other hand, we do not have time to dwell on such matters ahead of time, mulling them over, imagining any number of difficulties, becoming increasingly anxious and, possibly, fearing a worse worst than we need to. An example of which many of us probably have direct experience is when the anticipation of and waiting for an anxiety-provoking event (an operation perhaps, or a driving test, or a job interview) turns out to be significantly more stressful that the actual event itself.

When we apply a specifically life course focus to our consideration of stressful events, the timing of the experience in relation to normative life experiences also becomes important. For example, whilst we may all expect to experience bereavement at some point in our life, the death of a parent during our childhood is an 'off time' experience. As such, this adds an extra, but perhaps hidden, dimension to the stress of the event. Many of your younger clients will be experiencing levels of incapacity or disruption that are more usually associated with extreme old age. Likewise, their parents might have anticipated having to face serious heath issues in relation to their own parents, but not in relation to their children. The sense of disorientation that this can provoke stems from the contravention of our taken-for-granted expectations of how our life course would pan out. Both clients and their families may need to grieve for an imagined future that is now under threat and may not progress in the way they had anticipated.

Take some time now to complete Learning Task 5.1. It asks you to consider these various stress-enhancing conditions in relation to a number of clients you have worked with.

Learning Task 5.1   Stress-enhancing factors of life events

Think about two or three clients that you have worked with recently and note down in your Learning Journal what you believe to be the most stressful life event or transition they were each experiencing at the time.

Reflect on their experience in relation to the criteria typically associated with a higher rather than a lower experience of stress. Specifically, consider:

• To what extent was the event involuntary (i.e. imposed on the client) rather than voluntary (i.e. chosen)?

- Was the event anticipated? To what extent might the client have reasonably expected it to occur?
- To what extent did the event conform to normative expectations about its timing in relation to the client's age or life stage?
- How new and unfamiliar was the situation for the client? Had they had any prior direct or indirect experience of similar circumstances?
- How great was the change or adaptation demanded of the client in response to the event?
- How quickly did each client have to respond? Did they have time to reflect on their options, or were they under pressure to make important decisions within a limited timeframe?
- How predictable and certain was the outcome of the transition?

How do you think these factors affected the level and type of stress experienced by your clients?

Defining 'stress'

Since all life stages involve the management of change and transition, they also all involve the management of stress. But what do we mean by 'stress'? Before reading on, spend some time completing Learning Task 5.2.

Learning Task 5.2   What does 'stress' mean to me?

- Take a new page in your Learning Journal and a stopwatch (you will probably find the latter on the 'clock' section of your mobile phone menu).
- Set the timer on your stop watch for at least five minutes (10 would be better) and, in your Learning Journal, write whatever occurs to you in response to the opening phrase: *'The last time I was stressed* ....*'*
- Continue writing until the timer on your stopwatch indicates that time is up.
- Now, look back over what you have written and consider, preferably in discussion with at least one other person, what it suggests that 'stress' means to you.
- Can you come up with a (reasonably) concise definition of 'stress', say in fewer that 30 words?

Perhaps to an even greater degree than with regard to transitions and turning points, the topic of stress involves another plunge into the definitional quagmire, although in practice there is a degree of shared and taken-for-granted understanding as to what we mean by 'stress'. The likelihood is that, in Learning Task 5.2, the definition you came up with fell within one of two basic types: the first sees stress as a stimulus in the environment that impinges on the person and the second sees stress as a response within the person to circumstances that they find unpalatable.

The first type of definition, seeing stress in terms of the stimulus characteristics of the environment, constitutes something of an engineering or mechanistic perspective, and also represents our colloquial use of the term when we say 'I've been under a lot of stress lately' or 'I'm in a very high-stress job'. A key aspect of the environment that is typically considered to be stressful is major life events (for example job loss, bereavement or geographic relocation). This is the thinking that lies behind life event checklists such as Holmes and Rahe's (1967) Social Readjustment Rating Scale, where it is assumed that the greater the number and severity of disruptive events experienced by individuals in the previous one to two years, the greater is the likelihood that they will succumb to stress-related health problems. However, assigning fixed stress weightings to different life events is fraught with difficulty, and rescalings of the items in the Social Readjustment Rating Scale in 1977 and 1995 (Miller & Rahe, 1997) revealed a degree of variation in both the absolute level of stress accorded to some items and their perceived relative stressfulness. Marriage, for example, was given a lower stress rating than in the original study, whilst more anxiety than previously was expressed about the death of close friends, major illness, marital separation, mortgage foreclosure and work issues. As well as being susceptible to changes in our interpretation of the stressfulness of particular life events, such lists also fail to recognize individual differences in the impact and meaning of particular events for the individuals concerned. They should, therefore, be used with caution in client-centred practice, which gives primacy to clients' understanding of their situation.

Major life events are not the only stressful events in our environment. We can also be worn down by chronic conditions (for example impaired mobility, poor housing or chronic pain) and/or the accumulation of minor irritations or hassles (perhaps missing a bus, dropping a carton of milk and having a 'bad hair' day). Such events and experiences can contribute to the gradual erosion of our well-being. Because each individual event may not in isolation seem worth dwelling on, we frequently ignore them. Clients may not even think to mention minor difficulties with day-to-day tasks on the basis that they should just 'get on with life' and not bother about seemingly insignificant inconveniences. But such 'inconveniences' can, over time, mount into major stresses. Occupational therapists may be best placed amongst health and social care professionals to help in the relief of such aggravations.

The idea of stress being the accumulation of major life events, chronic conditions and/or day-to-day hassles represents the idea of stress as overload. Within this framework, stress is not our responsibility. It is something that happens to us. It is not our fault. It is encapsulated in a quotation cited by Cox (1985) from Sir Charles Symonds, a Ministry of Defence physician back in 1947, talking about psychological disorders in RAF flying personnel: 'it should be understood once and for all that stress is that which happens to the man, not that which happens in him; it is a set of causes, not a set of symptoms' (Symonds, 1947).

By way of contrast, the response model of stress defines 'stress' as the reaction of people's minds and bodies to demands placed upon them. It is a feeling of tension, anxiety or worry, as when we might say, 'I'm nervous about the presentation I have to give next week' or 'I always feel apprehensive and tongue-tied when talking to my doctor'. Its origins lie in studies of physiological responses to stressors, as in Selye's (1978) identification and account of the three-phase General Adaptation Syndrome, as described below:

1. An immediate *alarm reaction*, itself divided into two substages. The first substage (*shock*) involves a dip in the person's coping effectiveness (something Richard in our case study experienced on finding his mother lying on the floor after her CVA). The second substage is *counter shock* – the restitution and enhancement of coping effectiveness as the mobilized resources of the autonomic nervous system begin to have their effect.
2. A *resistance* stage, where people use a range of coping strategies to combat the response that the stressors have initiated.
3. A stage of *exhaustion and collapse* that is reached if the demands on the body are overwhelming or unremitting.

The elements of this sequence can be seen behaviourally in our case study, as we suggested above, in Richard's response to Helen's stroke. As his initial shock on finding his mother on the floor subsided, Richard embarked on a period of frantic, if not very effectual, rushing around, a desperate attempt 'to do something'. Then there followed a period of sustained, measured and effective management of the situation. Current exhaustion and despondency could well be the herald of collapse if preventive measures are not taken.

This emphasis on stress as a physiological response within the person is a perspective frequently adopted within health care settings, as, for example, when the website of the Health and Safety Executive (HSE; 2007) defines stress as 'the reaction people have to excessive pressure or other types of demands placed on them'. This is not, however, by any means the full story. It is not so much the actual level of pressure or demand that is important but rather the person's perception and interpretation of that pressure. In other words, rather than being either an environmental stimulus or an automatic response to the objective characteristics of a stressor, stress is best thought of as a process involving transactions between people and their environments, in which psychological processes within the person actively mediate between the stimulus and the response. This represents a third, and somewhat more sophisticated, notion of stress that is invoked, for example, when the HSE (2007) supplements its definition with the comment that stress arises when people 'worry that they can't cope'. Drawing on work from several sources (including Lazarus & Folkman, 1984; Cox, 1985; Lazarus, 1999), stress can be defined as those transactions which arise when people perceive that the demands, either real or imagined, of a situation exceed or severely tax their capacity – again, either perceived or imagined – to cope effectively. Thus, in our case study Sarah is concerned about whether the competing demands of a new baby and her career will exceed her capacity to cope. We can imagine that there may be several elements to this concern. It is likely, for example, that she is concerned about role overload. Will she and Ranjiv be able to make the necessary changes to their lifestyle that would make her combination of career and motherhood feasible? She may also be concerned about whether she has the necessary skills to care for an infant. Whilst she is close to her half-brother, Chris, she has limited direct experience of child care. As outsiders, we may think that her skills and experience as a nurse will stand her in good stead, but perhaps Sarah herself has not made this connection. Whatever the specifics of the situation, it should be clear that this transactional, or interactive, approach to conceptualizing stress immediately focuses attention on the individual's point of view. It prioritizes the person's appraisal of the situation over its objective characteristics. As such, it is consistent with the client-centred focus of health and social care practice.

The process model of stress directs attention to the cognitive appraisals (Lazarus & Folkman, 1984; Lazarus, 1999) made by individuals of both the situation they are in and their capacity to manage that situation. The first element of this process, or transaction – the primary appraisal – involves assessing the meaning of a particular situation to our well-being. We may decide one of three things: that it is irrelevant, that it is good (or positive) or that it is stressful. An assessment of 'stressful' triggers the secondary appraisal: an ongoing assessment of our resources for coping. Efforts to cope, successful or otherwise, are brought into play, and these processes influence our subsequent appraisal of the situation as stressful or not (Lazarus, 1999).

Pause for a few moments at this point to think about what an assessment of 'stressful' means. What thoughts, feelings and behaviours follow on from such an assessment? Learning Task 5.3 provides a structure for this reflection.

Learning Task 5.3   The symptoms of stress

- Think of a situation you recently found stressful (perhaps something that you wrote about in Learning Task 5.2).
- How did you know you were stressed? Make a list in your Learning Journal of your symptoms (i.e. the things you thought, felt and did that indicated you were stressed).
- Think more generally now about what other symptoms may be indicative of stress. Generate as long a list as possible. Don't worry about overlap; just try to get a sense of the range of symptoms that may be indicative of stress. If possible, generate this list in collaboration with two or three others so that you can build on and extend each others' ideas.
- When you have ground to a halt, look at your list and see to what extent you can organize this range of symptoms into groups. What would you call each group?

Discussions of the symptoms of stress generally distinguish, at the very least, between physiological, psychological and behavioural symptoms (for example Sutherland & Cooper, 1990). A more refined and nuanced classification is provided in the multimodal-transactional model of stress (Palmer & Dryden, 1995; Palmer, 1996). The seven response categories that it employs can be used by professionals wishing to undertake a comprehensive assessment of clients' responses to their situation.

Multimodal-transactional model of stress

Palmer and Dryden (1995; Palmer, 1996) have developed the cognitive appraisal (or transactional) model of stress to incorporate the seven categories, or modalities, that make up Lazarus's (1986, 1989) 'multimodal' model of personality.[1] These modalities are used as a framework for distinguishing and classifying different elements in the response to stress. The seven modalities, known collectively by the mnemonic BASIC-ID, are listed below, and the model is illustrated diagrammatically in Figure 5.1.

- *Behaviour:* overt behaviour that can be observed (e.g. driving erratically, restlessness, social withdrawal)
- *Affect:* emotions, moods and other strong feelings (e.g. anger, anxiety, fear)
- *Sensations:* physical sensations (e.g. dizziness, nausea, clammy hands)
- *Imagery:* vivid and/or recurring memories or imaginings (e.g. nightmares, flashbacks and memories of past failures)
- *Cognitions:* thoughts, opinions, judgements (e.g. 'I can't do this', 'It's not fair')
- *Interpersonal:* relationship factors (e.g. aggressive or passive interpersonal style, few social contacts)
- *Drugs/Biological:* drug use and health-related behaviours (e.g. smoking, lack of exercise, poor diet, alcohol abuse)

[1] In case it is causing confusion, we want to point out that there are two researchers named Lazarus cited in this chapter: Richard S. Lazarus, whose name is associated with the cognitive appraisal model of stress, and Albert A. Lazarus, whose multimodal theory of personality is incorporated into the multimodal-transactional model of stress.

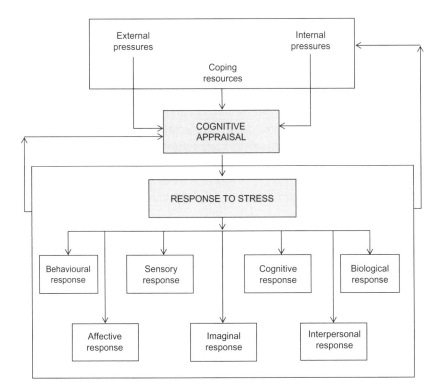

Figure 5.1 The multimodal transactional model of stress (Palmer & Dryden, 1995)
(Adapted with permission from SAGE Publications, London, Los Angeles, New Delhi and Singapore, from *Counselling for Stress Problems*, © S. Palmer & W. Dryden, 1995)

How many symptoms of stress or stress responses did you identify in Learning Task 5.2? Compare notes with a few colleagues and add up your grand total of symptoms and responses. When you realize that Palmer and Dryden (1995) distinguish over 140 different responses in their classification system, you will be aware of the myriad of ways in which stress can show itself. The symptoms/ responses that Palmer and Dryden identify, grouped under the BASIC-ID headings, are listed in Table 5.1. Look through this list in some detail. Which items did you identify whilst completing Learning Task 5.2? Which items did not occur to you? Did the ones you listed and the ones you omitted tend to fall within particular categories? How many of the stress responses can you identify in clients that you have worked with?

Table 5.1 Indicators of stress (Palmer & Dryden, 1995).

Behaviour	*Sensation* cont'd
alcohol/drug abuse	nausea
avoidance/phobias	tremors
increased nicotine/caffeine intake	aches/pains
restlessness	dizziness/feeling faint
loss of appetite/overeating	indigestion
anorexia, bulimia	premature ejaculation/
aggression/irritability	erectile dysfunction
poor driving	vaginismus/psychogenic
poor time management	dyspareunia
accident proneness	limited sexual and
impaired speech/voice tremor	sensual awareness
compulsive behaviour	butterflies in stomach
checking rituals	numbness
tics, spasms	dry mouth
nervous cough	cold sweat
low productivity	clammy hands
withdrawing from relationships	abdominal cramps
clenched fists	sensory flashbacks
teeth grinding	pain
type A behaviour	poor self-image
increased absenteeism	
decreased/increased sexual activity	*Imagery*
eating/walking/talking faster	Images of:
sulking behaviour	helplessness
frequent crying	isolation/being alone
unkempt appearance	losing control
poor eye contact	accidents/injury/failure
	humiliation/shame/embarrassment
Affect (emotions)	self and/or others dying/suicide
anxiety	physical/sexual abuse
depression	nightmares/distressing recurring dreams
anger	visual flashbacks
guilt	poor self-image
hurt	
morbid jealousy	*Cognitions*
shame/embarrassment	'I must perform well'
suicidal feelings	'Life should not be unfair'
	self/other damning statements
Sensation	low frustration statements, e.g.
tension	'I can't stand it'
headaches	'I must be in control'
palpitations	'It's awful, terrible, unbearable'
rapid heart beat	'I must have what I want'

Table 5.1   Continued

Cognitions cont'd	*Drugs/Biology*
'I must obey "my" moral codes and rules'	use of drugs, stimulants, alcohol, tranquillisers, hallucinogens
'Others must approve of me'	diarrhoea, constipation, flatulence
cognitive distortion, e.g. 'all or nothing' thinking	frequent urination
	allergies/skin rash
	high blood pressure/coronary heart disease (angina/heart attack)
Interpersonal	
passive/aggressive in relationships	dry skin
timid/unassertive	chronic fatigue/exhaustion/burnout
loner	cancer
no friends	diabetes
competitive	rheumatoid arthritis
puts others' needs before own	asthma
sycophantic behaviour	flu/common cold
withdrawn	lowered immune system
make friends with difficulty	poor nutrition, exercise and recreation
suspicious/secretive	organic problems
manipulative tendencies	biologically based mental disorders
gossiping	

(Adapted with permission from SAGE Publications, London, Los Angeles, New Delhi and Singapore, from *Counselling for Stress Problems*, © S. Palmer & W. Dryden, 1995)

The indicators of stress identified by Palmer and Dryden (1995) reflect automatic, negative, unchosen and unwelcome symptoms or outcomes of stress. They do not, however, need to be accepted as inevitable and unavoidable. Much can be done to overcome them, to reduce their severity and/or to replace them with more positive and constructive responses. In other words, much can be done to manage stress and its symptoms.

Managing stress

When we assess a situation as stressful, or when we experience unwelcome symptoms of stress, we make efforts, possibly very idiosyncratically, to cope. These efforts may be consciously and explicitly chosen, or they may be engaged in automatically without conscious thought. They may be effective or ineffective in improving the situation. They may even exacerbate it, in the long term if not immediately. In Learning Task 5.4, you are asked to consider the coping strategies of some of the people involved in our case study: what they did, how effective their efforts were and what else they might have done.

Learning Task 5.4 Efforts to cope

Think about two of the following people in the case study:

- Andrew
- Brian
- Mary
- Sarah

For each person, consider the following:

- What were the main stressors in the situation for them: major life changes, ongoing problematic situations, day-to-day hassles?
- What did they each do to cope with the stress?
- How effective were their efforts?
- What else might they have done to cope with the stress?
- How might you, as a health or social care professional, have helped them to modify their coping strategies for the better?

By 'coping' we mean the process of managing the external and/ or internal demands that strain or exceed our actual or perceived resources. This definition also describes a great deal of what is involved in managing life events; and all that is said in Chapter 3 under the 'Self', 'Support' and 'Strategies' categories of Goodman *et al.*'s (2006) '4-S' model is also applicable here. In the same way that a range of personal factors influence our capacity to manage life events, so, too, do these factors influence the coping resources and skills we can call upon in order to manage stress.

A commonly used classification of coping strategies (again deriving from the work of R. S. Lazarus and his colleagues) distinguishes between environment-focused and emotion-focused coping, categories that can be further subdivided. Thus, specific coping strategies can be grouped according to their more general function by distinguishing between four distinct goals: two directed at the environment (or situation) and two at the person (or self):

- *Environment* (or situation) focused coping, by:
  1. *Modifying the situation* and, thereby, the demands it makes on the individual, for example rescheduling appointments so that they coincide with bus timetables or providing equipment that makes the activities of daily living (such as dressing or cooking) easier.
  2. *Escaping from or avoiding the situation*, for example ending a stressful relationship, renegotiating responsibilities at work so they are compatible with current abilities or circumstances.
- *Person* (or self) focused coping, by:
  1. *Developing additional coping strategies or personal resilience*, for example attending classes in yoga, relaxation or assertion, developing new support systems.
  2. *Altering the way the situation is perceived and assessed*, for example reconsidering taken-for-granted goals, cognitive restructuring in order to challenge unrealistic expectations or irrational beliefs.

It is only the first of these categories (coping strategies that modifying the environment) that act directly on the situation making the demands. These strategies are aimed at altering or eliminating the source of life strains, and therefore represent the most direct way of coping with them. Attempts to resolve conflict through negotiation between the relevant parties would fall under this heading. However, in their study of responses to life strains Pearlin and Schooler (1978) found that such direct actions comprised the minority of coping responses, and offered four possible explanations for this. First, the individual may not recognize the situation as the source of the problem. Without this recognition, actions cannot consciously be mobilized towards altering it. Second, even if the source of the problem is recognized, people may lack the knowledge or skills, or indeed opportunity, to change it. Third, people may resist changing the situation out of fear that the resulting situation could be worse. And finally, the conditions producing the demands may be resistant and difficult to change, thus undermining motivation to try.

It is likely, therefore, that many people's efforts at coping will address the problem indirectly rather than directly. However, classifying particular coping strategies as serving particular functions is somewhat arbitrary in that a particular strategy may serve more than one function and/or its effect may change over time. For

example, developing assertion skills increases an individual's repertoire of coping skills (a person-focused function) and may make
them better able to negotiate a more satisfactory work role (an
environment-, problem- or task-focused function). Similarly, effective time management both enables us to cope more efficiently with
the demands placed upon us and changes the situation by reducing
the level of demand, and hence the amount of stress, we experience.
However, whilst, say, rescheduling the payment of bills may be an
effective short-term strategy for changing the situation, the bills do
all have to be paid in the end, and if the new schedule is not adhered
to the result may be an increase rather than a decrease in actual and
experienced level of stress. It has been suggested (Cox & Ferguson,
1991) that all coping serves one overall function: that of dealing
with the emotional correlates of stressful events and of creating a
sense of control.

Therefore, whilst the question of the relative effectiveness of different coping strategies is important, it is not necessarily easy to
answer. Most, if not all, strategies have their time and place, and,
indeed, effective coping inevitably involves the flexible utilization
of a range of strategies as demanded by the situation (Goodman
et al., 2006). Problem-focused strategies will be most appropriate
and tend to be most used in relation to aspects of the situation that
can be changed, whilst emotion-focused strategies can be more
effective when the situation is largely beyond the individual's
control, and must be adapted to rather than altered.

Interventions

Many interventions undertaken by those who work in health or
social care are designed to help clients who are finding that the
demands placed upon them tax or exceed their current resources.
In other words, many interventions we undertake are concerned
with the management of stress. An advantage of the BASIC-ID
framework is that, as well as being a framework for classifying
responses to stress, it can also be used as a basis for classifying and
choosing different approaches to stress management. It offers
the possibility of tailoring interventions effectively to meet the
particular needs of an individual client as reflected in his or her
stress response profile. Whilst, in their interventions, occupational

103

therapists emphasize activity and occupation, their work does, of course, engage all of the BASIC-ID modalities. Think about the interventions that you use with clients. Which modalities do they relate to? A number of possible intervention strategies that occupational therapists or other health and social care practitioners may use (based on Palmer, 1996, and grouped under the BASIC-ID modalities) are given in Table 5.2. These examples are only indicative – can you think of any others? Of course, many interventions will themselves be multimodal, involving several strategies that affect several BASIC-ID categories. Indeed, some individual strategies could be included under more than one heading. For example, working with clients to achieve a positive work–life balance could involve all or any of the BASIC-ID modalities.

Table 5.2 BASIC-ID groupings of possible occupational therapy interventions.

Behaviour	*Cognition*
Behaviour rehearsal	Challenging faulty inferences
Self-monitoring and recording	Challenging negative assumptions and thoughts
Empty chair	Positive self-statements
Exposure programme	Cognitive rehearsal
Skills development	Coping statements
Modelling	Problem-solving training
Paradoxical intention	Self-acceptance training
Therapeutic drama	Thought-stopping
Reinforcement programmes	Affirmations
Stimulus control	Accepting appropriate anxiety
Risk-taking exercises	
	Interpersonal
Affect	Assertion training
Anger expression/management	Communication training
Anxiety management	Contracting
Feeling identification	Social skills training
	Friendship/intimacy training
Sensation	Graded sexual approaches
Biofeedback	
Relaxation training	*Drugs/Biology*
Meditation	Self-care programmes
	Lifestyle changes (e.g. exercise regimes)
Imagery	Smoking-cessation programme
Positive imagery	Alcohol-reduction programme
Visualization	
Coping imagery	

Indicators of positive change can also be grouped under the BASIC-ID headings, and include the following:

- *Behaviour:* self-care rather than self-harm; substitution of constructive, appropriate behaviours for destructive, inappropriate behaviours; extinction of inappropriate behaviours
- *Affect:* awareness and acceptance of feelings
- *Sensation:* tension release; sensory pleasuring
- *Imagery:* coping images; positive changes in self-image
- *Cognition:* greater awareness; cognitive restructuring
- *Interpersonal:* non-judgemental acceptance of others; dispersal and avoidance of destructive, colluding relationships; use of constructive modelling
- *Drugs/biology:* better nutrition and exercise; cessation of substance abuse; use of appropriate medication where indicated.

It is also worth noting that, because it is grounded in the individual's personality and response to stress, rather than in the stressful situations themselves, the interventions listed in Table 5.2 are primarily focused on the person rather than the environment. Environment-focused strategies are largely concerned with modifying the immediate setting in which the client is embedded. The skill of the occupational therapist lies in flexibly and effectively blending both types of intervention according to clients' particular needs, preferences and circumstances. This emphasis is a crucial part of ethical, client-centred practice. Nonetheless, more broadly focused environmental interventions (for example working to increase the availability of resources or to change policies with regard to access to public transport) may also form a part of the health or social care professional's role. Again, it is a question of 'both/and' rather than 'either/or'.

Coping across the life course

There is limited evidence about how people's coping strategies change across the life course. What evidence there is suggests that changes in children's coping strategies are linked to cognitive developments, and that those changes in the strategies used by adults may tie in with the nature of the stress they experience and their interpretation of it. Thus, infants and very young children will try to manage the stress of a medical examination by trying to escape the situation and/or prevent the examination taking place (Hyson, 1983), at the same time giving vociferous vent to their feelings. During the years of childhood, however, they learn to use cognitive strategies for coping (Miller & Green, 1984; Brown *et al.*, 1986), for example distracting themselves by thinking of something else or making positive self-statements such as 'I can handle this' when about to undertake a stressful task.

In a study of age differences in stress and coping processes, Folkman *et al.* (1987) found that the middle-aged subjects tended to use more problem-focused approaches to coping, whereas the older subjects employed more emotion-focused strategies. The older subjects perceived, perhaps accurately (Pilgrim, 1997), their external stressors to be less changeable, making self-focused coping strategies seem more appropriate than situation-focused ones. It has been suggested (Pearlin & Skaff, 1996) that, with experience, people tend increasingly to rely on the management of the meaning of difficult situations rather than the management or change of the situations themselves. Whilst such evidence can inform our work with clients, suggesting what view of the situation our clients may be adopting, it is crucial that such general findings do not make us insensitive to the particular perspective of individual clients.

Before ending this chapter, we wish to reiterate how all of the points made about stress and its management apply to health and social care professionals as well as to their clients. It is important to acknowledge that all of us experience stress, and that this can be accentuated by working on a regular basis in responsible and demanding positions with others who are experiencing and vulnerable to stress. We therefore need to be aware of our own stress and our own coping strategies if we are to avoid burnout (Bassett & Lloyd, 2001; Painter *et al.*, 2003), and make the best possible therapeutic use of self. We have a responsibility to be fit to practise, and this includes taking continuing professional development and lifelong learning seriously. We need to put in place, and then use, personal strategies for managing our stress, and ensure that we are properly supported in our workplaces in this regard. These issues are addressed further in Chapter 9, the final chapter of this work book. Next, however, is one more chapter concerned with generic developmental tasks and skills. It considers strategies and interventions to promote effective decision-making, problem management and the development of new opportunities. This is followed by a chapter which considers how clients' experiences are put together in the form of a narrative. It is after this, in Chapter 8, that the experience of the occupational therapy practitioner takes centre stage.

6. *Planful Decision-making*

Every minute of every day we are immersed, whether we are aware of it or not, in a stream of decision-making. You can consider this further by turning to Learning Task 6.1, which will doubtless reveal that decision-making is a natural part of everyday life and that we make many different decisions on a daily basis.

Learning Task 6.1   Deciding what to do

In a day, we make dozens of decisions.

- Think about all the decisions you have made today. Jot them down in your Learning Journal, seeing how many you can identify. Here are a few likely ones to get you going:
  - What time to get up.
  - What to wear.
  - Whether to have breakfast.
  - What to have for breakfast.
  - Whether to brush your teeth.
  - Whether to read this book, and this chapter within this book.
  See how long you can make your list – go for quantity not quality at this stage.

It is likely that few, if any, of the items on your list will have been momentous decisions. To most of them you will have given only fleeting attention and, indeed, some might have been made so automatically that they hardly count as decisions; 'habits' may be a better definition of these sorts of decisions. However, perhaps within the last month, and almost certainly within the last year, you will have made

more momentous decisions in your personal, social, educational and/
or working life.

- Take a few moments to list some of the most significant decisions
  you have made in your life (perhaps turning back to the transitions
  exercise in Chapter 4 for inspiration) and, for good measure, add
  those you envisage making over the next two to three years.
  ○ How did you approach making these decisions? Were they made
    quickly or did you linger over them? How much thought did
    you give to them? Who influenced you in your decision-making?
    What feelings were involved?
  ○ With hindsight, how do you think your decision-making strate-
    gies could have been improved?

Learning Task 6.1 encourages you to think not only about *what*
decisions you have made but also about *how* you made them. The
chances are that the different approaches or styles of decision-
making which you have used, possibly in combination, fall into the
following three categories:

1. *Intuitive/emotional:* going with your 'gut reaction'; making
   decisions, often spontaneously, on the basis of what 'feels
   right'.
2. *Compliant:* deferring to others' choices, possibly because you
   see them as experts, because the decision is not very important
   to you or because you wish to please the other people
   involved. This, in effect, involves allowing others to decide for
   you.
3. *Planful:* exploring your needs, situation and options, then choosing on the basis of a weighing-up of the costs and benefits of each
   alternative.

It is likely that your use of these strategies has ranged from confident to hesitant.

Most significant decisions are planned at least to some degree:
we assess the situation and our options, and then choose and execute
one line of action. However, we do not necessarily complete each
of these tasks thoroughly or effectively, and, indeed, may not really
be aware of the process we are using. Guidelines designed to direct

and improve our decision-making, including the framework presented in the following section, represent efforts to make explicit and refine this process. Whilst planful decision-making has much to recommend it, this does not mean that all decisions require you to plod methodically through all options and stages to reach one. There are occasions when intuitive/emotional and compliant decisions may be appropriate (although, ideally, we should use these strategies knowingly rather than by default, that is we should decide to use an intuitive or compliant style). Thus, intuitive decisions may be useful in situations where time is at a premium (Carnall, 2007) or, for example, in emergencies, or in the face of unforeseen opportunities. Compliant decisions can save not only time but energy and effort as well. This may indicate a deferral to the greater knowledge or expertise of others, or may, in group situations, be taken in the spirit of compromise. A balanced decision will frequently include elements of all three decision styles.

Problem management and opportunity development

Decision-making is not an end in itself. We make decisions for a purpose. Frequently, the purpose of decision-making is to solve a problem (which could be very minor, for example what snack to have when we are hungry in the middle of the afternoon, or very major, as, for example, the decision that Andrew in our case study, pp. 6–11, has to make about his future after graduation). However, in the same way that stress cannot always be completely eradicated (see Chapter 5) so problems cannot always be solved. Very often problems are managed rather than resolved, with compromise, balance and the reconciliation of conflicting factors being the order of the day. The framework described in this section offers strategies for finding this middle ground, and is described, therefore, as a model of problem management rather than of problem-solving. Portraying situations as 'problems' goes somewhat against the current zeitgeist of positive thinking, with its focus on possibilities rather than constraints, and, in keeping with this, the model can also be seen as a sequence of strategies designed to facilitate the exploration, development and taking-up of opportunities, allowing it to go by the acronym PMOD (problem management and opportunity development).

It is unlikely that the model discussed below is totally unfamiliar to you. As already indicated, it describes a process that most of us engage in, perhaps not in its entirety, and perhaps implicitly rather than explicitly, in the course of our daily lives. It is also likely that many of you will have come across one or more versions of this process in more formal settings, perhaps as part of career exploration workshops or as a basis for personal target setting in end-of-year self-assessments. It is a very useful framework for planning work with clients, and indeed is implicit in the therapeutic process (Hagedorn, 2002). In an initial interview with a client, we aim to understand the current position, exploring the situation and focusing on the relevant areas for intervention. Subsequently, we decide with the client on appropriate goals, taking stock of the possible ways of achieving them and selecting the best way of doing so. We then help the client to put the plan into action and, as it proceeds, we continually monitor and assess progress until the situation has been managed appropriately. This is the underlying framework for all work with clients, and for most of us it is so familiar that we are not conscious that we are working to it – it is part of our tacit knowledge and understanding (Hagedorn, 2002; Findlay, 2004).

The version presented below, derived from Egan and Cowan (1979), is designed to be as comprehensive in scope as possible. It describes the process of effective problem management and opportunity development in four stages, each with two substages, or steps, making eight steps in all, as summarized in Box 6.1. Not all eight steps will require equal amounts of attention, and some are likely to be considerably easier than others. This will, of course, vary across individuals and situations. When using the model as a framework for work with clients, it is also important to remember that clients may not need your input with every step. Your interventions may dip in and out of the sequence, with clients addressing the tasks in some of the steps in their own way, either on their own or with other people in their support convoy. At some points you may be a major resource for clients, and at others you may be more a source of reassurance and support. Remember, however, discussions in Chapter 2 about your location on a client's support convoy. By virtue of the role-dependent nature of your relationship with clients, there is a limit to how close to the core of their personal convoy you can, or should, get.

Box 6.1 Steps in the process of problem management and opportunity development

Stage 1: Situational review: understanding the current scenario.
        Step 1a: Exploration
        Step 1b: Focusing
Stage 2: Planning where to get to (ends): defining the preferred scenario.
        Step 2a: Reframing
        Step 2b: Establishing goals
Stage 3: Deciding what to do (means): developing a clear plan of action.
        Step 3a: Census of options
        Step 3b: Programme choice
Stage 4: Words into deeds: implementing plans and evaluating progress.
        Step 4a: Implementation
        Step 4b: Evaluation

The core of the PMOD model rests on the proposition that the most effective decision-making, problem management and opportunity development address four fundamental and progressive issues: understanding the current scenario, defining the preferred scenario, developing a clear plan of action, and implementing plans and evaluating progress. Each of these stages can be divided into two steps which reflect, first, a period of exploration, data collection and opening-up of the issue, and, second, a period of decision-making and careful, focused assessment. The model bears many similarities to the model for which Egan is most widely known, that of the skilled helper (Egan, 2007), save that it places 'action' (in the form of implementation and evaluation) as a distinct final stage rather than, or perhaps as well as, a stream that runs through all stages in the process.

Stage 1: Situational review: understanding the current scenario

A common catchphrase that sums up the rationale for systematic decision-making and planning is 'If you don't know where you're going, you'll probably end up somewhere else'. Think about this for a while. It implies that you have expectations and assumptions, even if you have not put them into words, and that you may well be surprised (and perhaps disconcerted) if these expectations, which you were not really even aware you had, are confounded. This is what happens when our experience does not conform to our assumptions about the way the world works and the 'normal, expectable life course'. This, of course, happens for nearly all our clients and for the people in our case study. It follows from this that the place to start when trying to help clients take control of their decision-making (or, indeed, take control of our own decision-making process) is to undertake a comprehensive review of the current situation. This constitutes Step 1a in the decision-making process: *Exploration*.

Step 1a is generally triggered by awareness of the necessity for making a decision. It involves collecting data and resisting the temptation to dash into the first course of action that occurs to us. It is to some extent analogous to the contemplation stage in Prochaska *et al.*'s (1992) cycle of intentional change model considered in Chapter 3, and it involves examining the life space and asking questions such as 'What is going on?' and 'What problems, issues, concerns or undeveloped opportunities are there now or on the horizon?'

Most reviews of the personal life space reveal a complex scenario with many varied, multifaceted and contradictory elements. There is too much to deal with all at once, and so we must decide where to direct our energies first. This constitutes Step 1b: *Focusing*, and it shares similarities with Prochaska *et al.*'s (1992) preparation stage.

The general point is that Step 1b represents a decision-making stage based on the data collected during Step 1a. On occasions, it is relatively easy to decide where to focus first. Some particular element in the life space may seem an obvious, logical and worthwhile place to start. However, in other instances there may be many pressing issues, all of which seem equally important. Principles for guiding the decision about where to focus first include:

- As a priority, work to *defuse any crises*.
- Begin with an issue that is a *major concern*.
- Begin with a *manageable task or issue*.
- Address an issue that, if managed, will *lead to some general improvement* in the person's assessment of the quality of his or her life space.
- Start with something the person is *willing to work on*.
- Start with something that is *under the person's control*.
- Select an issue where *the benefits of resolving it outweigh the costs*.

113

Think about these criteria in relation to Brian's initial response to his sister's CVA. Whilst all the activities he undertook or considered may well be important at some stage, it is questionable whether they were the most appropriate place to start or whether they made the most effective use of his time and skills. Arguably, his organizational skill could have been used to greater effect if he had spent time checking whether Mary, his mother, needed any practical assistance (with transport to the hospital, for example) or possibly arranging for someone to look after Wicket the dog.

Stage 2: Planning where to get to (ends): defining the preferred scenario

In Stage 1 we work with clients, first, to explore and clarify their own understanding of their current situation and, then, having reviewed the issues that need to be addressed, we reach a decision about where to begin. Having a clear insight into our current situation, and being well aware of what is most in need of immediate attention, does not, however, mean that we necessarily know what we should do about it. Whereas Stage 1 is about understanding the situation as it is, Stage 2 in the PMOD model is about developing a vision of how the situation could be different. This frequently requires that clients move beyond their current world view and develop new and different images of possible futures. This is the purpose of Step 2a: *Reframing*. We look to the future and ask: 'What do we need or want in place of what we currently have?' and 'How would things look if they were better?' Through the use of creative techniques (see Box 6.2 for a couple of examples), clients can be encouraged to develop new perspectives that take them beyond their current world view and into new, unconsidered possibilities. As more possible futures are discovered, the options for goal selection increase, and the database for selecting the most suitable goals is enhanced.

Box 6.2   Techniques for promoting creativity

Two widely used techniques for promoting creativity – the first verbal and the second visual – are *creative idea generation* (or *thought showering*) and *mind mapping*.

- *Creative idea generation*

  Creative idea generation is a process, first documented as *brain-storming* in the 1930s (Osborn, 1963), designed to generate the maximum number of ideas relating to a particular issue or area of interest. It is based on four key principles, or rules:

  ○ *A focus on quantity:* The focus is on generating as many ideas as possible in order to provide the largest possible pool of alternatives. In groups, people call out all and any ideas about the topic that come into their heads, however bizarre they may initially appear. This is based on the assumption that quantity breeds quality and so a scribe records every suggestion made.

  ○ *The postponement and withholding of judgement:* Fear of criticism can make people reluctant to contribute, and ruling it out at this stage can help create a supportive and playful atmosphere, where everyone is keen to make suggestions and anything is assumed to be possible.

  ○ *The building on each other's ideas:* Whilst individuals can engage in creative idea generation on their own, it works best when it is the joint effort of at least two people who can then build on or expand each other's suggestions.

  ○ *The encouragement of wild and unusual suggestions:* Associations between the suggestions are often made quite subconsciously, as in the word-association game 'tennis, elbow, foot', and this can lead to the generation of unusual suggestions that would probably not have emerged through the use of more logical, rational thought. These leaps of imagination can open up new possibilities and ways of thinking that may lead ultimately to more creative solutions.

  Only after the process of idea generation is exhausted are the suggestions assessed and a selection made from among them.

  In terms of our case study, this technique may help Helen identify and then choose between possible ways of maintaining her involvement in gardening whilst she is unable to participate actively; and it may help Andrew think creatively about his options after graduating.

- *Mind mapping*

  Mind maps (Buzan, 2002), or spidergraphs, are visual representations of thoughts relating to a particular idea, problem or topic and the links between them. Mind mapping, like the process of life space mapping discussed in Chapter 2, is a technique that uses visual means to investigate and develop associations with and ramifications of a key issue or question. Working alone or with others, the subject to be considered is written or depicted diagrammatically in the centre of a page. Then, using colour, writing and/or drawing, lines are drawn from the central subject to other words, ideas or images that spring from it. Links between different elements of the mind map can be explored and indicated. When the subject and associations are exhausted, the ideas can be followed up, discarded and organized as seems best.

Here is an example of a mind map that Andrew could use to try to think about whether or not to go to the United States. Once completed, Andrew could look at his feelings and ideas, and work out a course of action or choose consciously to delay the decision for the moment (ideally setting a time when he will reconsider the matter).

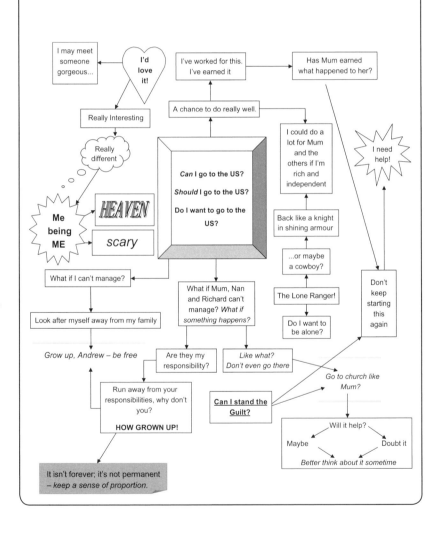

Step 2a is a divergent phase: a phase of opening up and data collection, with the result that the preferred scenarios may at this point in time be couched in fairly general, impressionistic terms. Like Step 1a, it is followed by a convergent phase: a phase of closing down and decision-making. This is Step 2b: *Establishing goals*. Some clients, once they have developed more ideas about their situation, may be clear about what best to do to move towards achieving it. Others may need help, education and support in the process of goal-setting. You may well be familiar with one or more of the not dissimilar acronyms that aim to describe the quality of useful goals, for example SMART (specific, measurable, adequate, realistic, time-bounded). Box 6.3 summarizes, and elaborates upon, these characteristics.

Box 6.3   Characteristics of useful goals

Useful goals tend to have the following characteristics:

- they are *behavioural* (i.e. concrete, clear and specific)
- they are *relevant* to the desired future scenario
- they are *adequate* (i.e. capable of promoting substantial movement towards the desired outcome)
- they are *realistic* (i.e. capable of being accomplished within the available resources)
- they are under the *control* of the client rather than someone else
- they are *valued* by the client
- progress towards them is *measurable*
- *criteria* indicating their accomplishment can be established
- they are *time-bounded* in that a realistic timeframe for their accomplishment is indicated

Think about Andrew and Sarah in the case study. To what extent do their goals meet these criteria?

Even when goals with the qualities listed in Box 6.3 have been established, the precise ways in which they could be best accomplished may not be clear. Goals are the ends to which the client is working. Stage 3 in the problem management and opportunity development process involves developing the means, the specific programmes, for achieving them.

Stage 3: Deciding what to do (means): developing a clear plan of action

Whereas Stages 1 and 2 are concerned with scenarios: 'Where am I now?' and 'Where do I want to get to?' Stage 3 is concerned with strategies: 'What do I need to do to move from the current to the preferred scenario?' and 'What would be the best package of strategies?' Nonetheless, the pattern of alternating opening-up and closing-down steps continues, with Step 3a involving the exploration of possible courses of action: a *census of options*. As with Step 2a (*Reframing*), this requires creativity, and, again, the techniques of creative idea generation or mind mapping can be used to generate ideas, possibilities and alternative courses of action.

In advocating the use of the problem management and opportunity development sequence, it is important to remember that it is a series of guidelines which must always be used mindfully and flexibly when working with individual clients. It is not a set of rules to be applied rigidly. Thus, whilst many of us tend to engage in too limited an exploration of possible alternatives at this stage, as Mary did in our case study, it is also possible to gather more information than is required to make a good decision. It is not necessary, for example, for prospective students to visit every university in the country that offers occupational therapy in order to decide which to put down on their UCAS form. The decision is important, but can be made on less information than is theoretically available.

We need to think about what type of outcome we should be striving for; it is not necessary, feasible or desirable to throw all our resources at every decision. The most suitable approach to decision-making depends on what type of outcome you are seeking. Strategies to choose between include *optimizing*, *satisficing*, *maximax* and *maximin*.

- *Optimizing:* where the strategy is to choose the best possible solution from the maximum range of options. The feasibility and, indeed, the appropriateness of optimizing is influenced by the importance of the decision, the time available for solving it, the cost (time and emotional costs, as well as financial) associated with different alternatives, available external resources and personal resources and values. For important and major life decisions, this is the preferred strategy, and is the goal of most decision-making guidelines. It is generally, however, an aspiration rather than an achievement since there are constraints of time, information, resources, motivation and/or energy, which nearly always apply.

- *Satisficing:* where the first or most readily available 'good enough' alternative is chosen, rather than searching out and waiting for the best possible solution. The term 'satisficing' is an amalgam of the words 'satisfactory' and 'sufficient' and describes a strategy appropriate for many small and routine decisions, for example where to park, what shirt to wear, which pen to use.
- *Maximax:* where the goal is to 'maximize the maximums'. It involves 'reaching for the sky', and choosing the option that offers the most favourable possible outcome, irrespective of the effort or difficulties involved. It is the strategy to choose when risk-taking is acceptable and failure can be countenanced.
- *Maximin:* where, by 'maximizing the minimums', the option chosen is that with the least possible negative outcome. It is a low-risk strategy ('a bird in the hand is worth two in the bush') and is appropriate where the consequences of failure are particularly harmful or undesirable.

Gathering too much information can lead to several problems (Harris, 1998):

- *Decision delay:* the time required to obtain and process the information can result in the decision being continually put off whilst more and more material is collected. A decision may be given more attention than it warrants, and a decision for which there was originally no time pressure may become urgent. The decision-making, or rather the lack of it, can also become a reason for not doing other important things.
- *Information overload:* the amount of information may be too much for the individual to manage and assess properly. Some, possibly important, material will be forgotten.
- *Selective use of information:* the decision-maker, overwhelmed by the amount of material available, may flee to the familiar and attend only to that which supports preconceived ideas. Creativity will thereby be inhibited.
- *Mental fatigue:* exhaustion can lead to slower, poorer-quality decision-making.
- *Decision fatigue:* ground down by the need to make a seemingly unending stream of decisions, the person can tire, leading to fast,

119

ill-considered choices or decision paralysis (i.e. the inability to make any decisions at all).

Having generated a list of alternative courses of action, a selection must be made from among them and a detailed plan drawn up of how to implement them. This is Step 3b: *Programme choice*, and, as with Steps 1b and 2b, is a decision-making or closing-down phase. Basically, the task is to (1) organize the alternatives generated in Step 3a around some central themes, (2) using these themes as a guide, arrange the alternatives into different possible packages of ways forward and (3) choose the course of action that best fits (in the broadest sense of the word) the client's needs. This process can be greatly assisted by using the technique of force-field analysis (see Learning Task 6.2).

Learning Task 6.2   Force-field analysis

Force-field analysis (see, for example, Hopson & Scally, 1999) is a technique designed to improve your chances of achieving an objective you have set yourself. It recognizes (like Prochaska *et al.*'s (1992) cycle of intentional change model) that there is a world of difference between commitment to action and actual enactment. It is a technique to use when you have a clear idea of what you want to achieve and how you could go about achieving it. It helps you to explore systematically those factors that will help or hinder your achievement of your goals. Furthermore, it can help maintain and revive motivation in the face of disappointments, hurdles, loss of momentum and apathy.

FORCE-FIELD ANALYSIS

The basic premise of force-field analysis is that a problematic situation can be thought of as a state of equilibrium between the forces for change (i.e. facilitating forces) and the forces resisting change (i.e. restraining forces), as illustrated below.

The identification of these forces, their direction (that is for or against the desired change), their strength and how they can be modified is the 'field of forces' that the technique seeks to 'analyse'.

Your task is to use this procedure to explore a goal you or a client is currently facing and to use the action plan that it generates as a mechanism for monitoring progress.

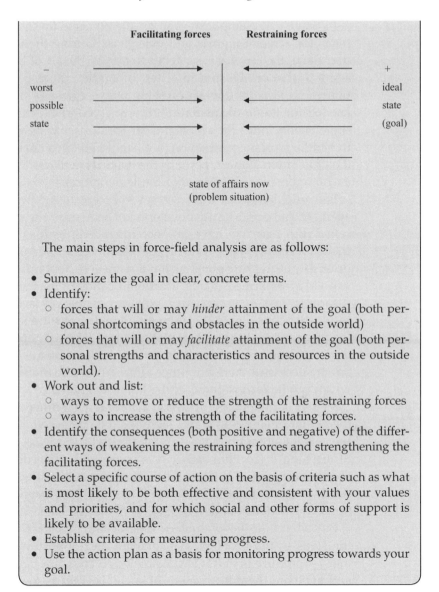

The main steps in force-field analysis are as follows:

- Summarize the goal in clear, concrete terms.
- Identify:
  - forces that will or may *hinder* attainment of the goal (both personal shortcomings and obstacles in the outside world)
  - forces that will or may *facilitate* attainment of the goal (both personal strengths and characteristics and resources in the outside world).
- Work out and list:
  - ways to remove or reduce the strength of the restraining forces
  - ways to increase the strength of the facilitating forces.
- Identify the consequences (both positive and negative) of the different ways of weakening the restraining forces and strengthening the facilitating forces.
- Select a specific course of action on the basis of criteria such as what is most likely to be both effective and consistent with your values and priorities, and for which social and other forms of support is likely to be available.
- Establish criteria for measuring progress.
- Use the action plan as a basis for monitoring progress towards your goal.

Stage 4: Words into deeds: implementing the plan and evaluating progress

The final stage in the problem management and opportunity development procedure is the most action-oriented of the stages and addresses the issues of 'Putting my action plans into practice' and 'How well am I doing?' Its first step (Step 4a) is *Implementation*.

In Stage 3 the emphasis was on the *strategy*, that is the overall plans for achieving goals and objectives. During the implementation stage, the emphasis switches to *tactics* (the art of being able to adapt a plan on the spot in order to handle unforeseen complications) and *logistics* (the art of being able to provide the resources needed for the implementation of any given plan). It may be that some clients, once they have a clear idea of what they need to do to handle a problem situation, are able to go ahead and undertake it on their own. Others, perhaps the majority, will need support and encouragement at this stage of implementation.

Force-field analysis traverses several steps in the problem management and opportunity development sequence, and can again be called into play. We have all encountered difficulties as we have tried to execute plans, but the completion of a force-field analysis prior to putting our plans to the test means, hopefully, that 'forewarned is forearmed'. Thus, the identification of 'restraining forces' (Learning Task 6.2) serves to highlight possible obstacles, with the result that consideration can be given ahead of time to difficulties that may arise at the implementation stage. Furthermore, the census of options that comprises Step 3a means that if some action plans are unsuccessful there are other alternatives already on the books which can be reconsidered in the light of experience.

Step 4a is an opening-up phase in a somewhat different way from the earlier opening-up steps. Here the data collected are not about the current situation (as in 1a), the desired future (2a) or the ways of reaching it (3a), but rather it is concerned with collecting data about the practicality and effectiveness of converting words into deeds. It leads into the final step in the problem management and opportunity development model, Step 4b: *Evaluation*.

But what is to be evaluated? One benefit of clearly delineating the steps in the problem management and opportunity development procedure is that it is possible to go back through each stage and evaluate the effectiveness of each. This leads to four general questions:

- *How effective was the implementation?* Did the client do what they had planned to do? This assesses the quality of their *participation* and is, in effect, an evaluation of Step 4a.
- *Did the action plan lead to the expected outcome?* Did the client's participation in the action plan move them significantly closer to reaching their goal? This assesses the degree of *effectiveness* of the

particular programme chosen. It is, in effect, an evaluation of Stage 3.

• *Has the 'preferred scenario' become a reality?* Is the client's current life space closer to their ideal than previously? This assesses the degree of *goal achievement*, and is an evaluation of Stage 2 of the problem management and opportunity development sequence.

• *Has the original problem or dilemma been eased?* Is the original situation that prompted the problem management and opportunity development procedure being managed more effectively than previously? This assesses *need fulfilment*: the extent to which the client's needs have been met. It is an evaluation of Stage 1 and is the ultimate question since it deals with the reason for starting the problem management and opportunity development procedure in the first place.

Evaluation requires that clients assess their achievements and compare them with the criteria that have emerged out of the systematic use of the problem management and opportunity development procedure. It enables both client and therapist to determine whether and what further work needs to be done, or whether the client's needs have been sufficiently met for their relationship to terminate, at least for the present.

To recap: the PMOD procedure is a sequence of four stages, each comprising two steps: first, an opening-up step that involves collecting various types of data and, second, a closing-down step that involves making decisions on the basis of that data. A risk in all stepwise presentations of sequences is that the processes may appear to be more linear and one-directional than is the case. Whilst the model itself is linear, and the process is linear in the sense that, by the end, the person will have moved from Step 1a through Stages 1, 2, 3 and 4 to Step 4b, there is much moving back and forth between different stages. The boundaries between different stages tend to be blurred. Furthermore, there is no assumption that each step will be of equal significance or duration. In other words, all the caveats that apply to the model of transition dynamics also apply here.

A number of other characteristics of the PMOD model warrant attention. It is worth noting that, in two different ways, the model is cumulative. First, the stages are cumulative in that, generally speaking, later stages are successful only to the extent that earlier stages have also been successfully addressed. A frequent mistake in problem management and opportunity development is attempting to begin too far along the sequence, for example taking the first course of action that occurs to us, without thinking of whether there may be more suitable alternatives or whether it really will address the issue we are concerned about. Several characters in the case study (Mary and Brian, for instance) either fell into this trap or were tempted to. Second, the model is also cumulative in the sense that the skills needed for each stage build on those needed for the previous stage. Thus, the skills needed for achieving the goals of Stage 2 include those needed to achieve the goals of Stage 1, plus some more. The skills needed for Stage 3 include those needed for Stages 1 and 2, plus some more again. And so on.

This chapter has outlined key dimensions in the task of problem management and opportunity development. As already suggested, it covers similar issues and concerns to Prochaska *et al.*'s (1992) cycle of intentional change model. Learning Task 6.3 invites you to consider this in more detail.

Learning Task 6.3 Comparing the cycle of intentional change model and the PMOD framework

Both the stages of intentional change (Prochaska *et al.*, 1992) and the PMOD framework (Egan & Cowan, 1979) are concerned with the process of deciding on, planning, implementing and evaluating change.

For this learning task, you should review these two models, and then consider and make notes on their similarities and differences.

The stages in these models are listed below as an aide-memoire, but you should refer back to Chapter 3 and/or to earlier sections of this chapter as necessary.

Stages of Intentional Change

Precontemplation
Contemplation
Preparation
Action
Maintenance

Problem Management and Opportunity Development

Situational review (Exploration and focusing)
Defining preferred scenarios (Reframing and establishing goals)
Developing an action plan (Option census and programme choice)
Action (Implementation and evaluation)

We close this section by reiterating that the PMOD framework is a set of guidelines, not a set of procedures and strategies written in stone. There is, as the saying goes, more than one way to skin a cat. It is something to take with you into your practice and use flexibly, critically and mindfully. For the moment, think about one of the case study characters, possibly Richard, Helen's younger son, and consider how the use of the PMOD framework could help him to make a decision about his plans for the next few years.

Decision-making in a life course context

Living involves growth and change, and, no matter how good our decision-making skills are, and no matter how appropriate the decisions are that we make at any particular point in time, the future holds twists and turns which we cannot predict and which render our decisions out of date or even obsolete. This is, after all, the essence of the view, presented in Chapter 2, of the life course as an alternating sequence of structure-changing and structure-building phases. While the decisions we make in adjusting to changing life events may be tackled separately, each decision is actually a link in a long chain of choices. Each decision we make builds on our previous decisions and in turn stimulates and influences our future decisions. In looking at a particular decision, it is important to distinguish between the *decision process* and the *decision outcome* (Carnall, 2007). The decision-making process is irreversible in the sense that time cannot be reversed. It propels us forward through a series of decision steps. The outcome of our decisions – the actions we take and their consequences – often can be changed by making new decisions as new alternatives become available.

Every opportunity developed, every problem solved or managed and every decision made occurs within the individual's life space, the crucial concept for analysing and understanding the person in a life course context. Decisions are made within a decision environment: 'the collection of information, alternatives, values and preferences available at the time of the decision' (Harris, 1998, p. 2). This environment influences and constrains the quality of the decision that can be made. The decision environment rarely, if ever, includes all possible information (all of it accurate) about every possible alternative. Time constraints often mean that a decision needs to be made within a particular timeframe, irrespective of whether all the potentially relevant information is available. Even with unlimited time, it may not be possible to gather full information about, or even identify, all alternatives. And even if such detail were available, it might well bring with it all the problems of information overload. Helping clients to make, act on and evaluate decisions is ultimately concerned with the art of the possible.

7. *Telling Tales*

It is not unusual for questions that seemingly ask for short, straight-forward answers actually to generate lengthy, convoluted responses (Riessman, 2002). Most of us, when invited to talk about an aspect of our life course, will tell a story rather than divide our experience into clear, unambiguous categories. You will find this with clients, especially as you develop a close working relationship with them. They want you to understand a meaningful whole, not simply respond to a detached, impersonal list of facts, symptoms or problems.

As authors of our life story, we select from our countless daily experiences what to include and what to omit. We weave what we select into a narrative, and link what is happening now with what has passed, and what may happen in the future. Thus, the experiences that Andrew, from our case study (pp. 6–11), chooses to focus on in his life story will both influence and be influenced by what he decides to do on graduation from university. You will find that your clients will, on the one hand, make choices that fit in with their current understanding of their life structure or personal narrative and, on the other hand, adjust their stories to accommodate their new experiences and decisions. This is an important aspect of dealing with new events.

Recognition of the significance of this human tendency to strive to place experiences into a wider and coherent story has led to a 'narrative turn' in many health-related disciplines and professions, including medicine (Hunter, 1991; Hyden, 1997; Greenhalgh & Hurwitz, 1998), nursing (Sandelowski, 1991), psychiatry and psychotherapy (Brown *et al.*, 1996) and occupational therapy (Mattingly, 1998; Clouston, 2004). Narrative theorists of the life course (for example Cohler, 1982; McAdams, 1997; Cohler &

Hostetler, 2003) focus on the process of reinterpreting the past in order to develop and maintain a coherent story. The narrative perspective emphasizes 'emplotment': the process of casting oneself as the main character in a narrative that is meaningful, productive and fulfilling (Cochran, 1997). This stance is resonant with the way in which occupational therapists work with clients to create and negotiate a constructive plot structure within clinical time that places therapeutic actions within a larger therapeutic story (Mattingly, 1994). Several frameworks for distinguishing and analysing 'illness narratives' have been identified (Frank, 1995; Hyden, 1997; Crossley, 2000; Ezzy, 2000; Bury, 2001).

Narrative characteristics

A narrative, or story, offers a way of making sense of our experiences by ordering them in a sequence across time, according to a theme (Bruner, 1990, 1991). If events are described randomly, they are likely to make little sense, and so a requirement of even the simplest coherent narrative is that it has, like a life, a beginning, a middle and an end. From any one set of life experiences more than one story could be told, and accounts of the life course reflect decisions made concerning which events are sufficiently significant to include, what themes best provide a coherent and meaningful plot, and the degree and type of closure given to the story (Murray, 1986). A life story can be represented graphically, as explored in Learning Task 7.1.

Learning Task 7.1   Lifeline

Turn to a blank sheet in your Learning Journal and, using the page horizontally rather than vertically, allow the left- and right-hand edges of the page to represent the beginning and end of your life respectively and draw, in the manner of a temperature chart, a line across the page to depict the peaks and troughs experienced in your life so far, and those you would predict for the future.

- When you have finished, sit back and ask yourself some questions about this graph (your 'lifeline'): What is its general shape? Does it continue to rise throughout life? Does it depict peaks and troughs around some arbitrary mean? Alternatively, is there a plateau and subsequent fall in the level of the curve? Is it punctuated with major or only relatively minor peaks and troughs?

- The horizontal axis represents time; but how about the vertical axis: what dimension does that reflect?
- What (or who) triggered the peaks and troughs in the graph? Why did they occur at the time that they did?
- What might have been done (or was done) to make the peaks higher and the troughs shallower? How may the incidence and height of the peaks be increased in the future? And the incidence and depth of the troughs decreased?
- What positive results emerged from the troughs and what were the negative consequences of the peaks?

The same life story can be told in many different ways. Consider this by examining your lifeline and think about how you would describe it differently depending on your reason for telling it, and who you were telling it to. Ask yourself, for example:

- What would the similarities and difference be between the account of your educational and/or work history that you would give to an old family friend you had not seen for several years and to a prospective employer during a job interview?
- To what extent and in what ways do you tell different versions of significant life events to members of your family and to your closest friends? Try to think of some specific examples of when you have done this. Was one version more 'true' than the other, or was each, in its own way, equally true?

Think about and, ideally, discuss with colleagues how clients could be motivated to tell their life story in a particular way to you as a health and social care practitioner. Does this matter? What, if anything, should you do about it?

Perhaps most crucially, narrative construction provides a mechanism for developing and maintaining a sense of identity. However, the capacity to understand and mould our life in story form emerges only gradually. Dan McAdams, a major theorist in this area, proposes that the key structural elements making up a personal narrative develop sequentially and cumulatively across a person's life. These elements, and the timetable of their emergence, are summarized in Table 7.1.

Table 7.1 The emergence of key structural elements of a life story (McAdams, 1997).

Life stage	Emerging narrative element
Infancy	*Narrative tone:* a general sense of optimism or pessimism that pervades a person's narrative.
Pre-school years	*Personal imagery:* memorable images of a particular episode, combining feelings, knowledge and inner sensations.
Childhood	*Thematic lines:* recurrent patterns reflecting what the characters in a narrative want and how they pursue their objectives over time.
Late adolescence	*Ideological settings:* a set of beliefs about what is right and true.
Young adulthood	*Characters (or imagoes):* internalized complexes of actual or imagined persons.
Middle adulthood	*Generative denouement:* an envisioned ending to one's personal narrative that allows some aspect of the self to live on.
Late adulthood	*Narrative evaluation:* the review, evaluation, reconciliation to and acceptance of our life story.

The seeds of our personal narrative are sown, suggests McAdams, during the first year of life, and throughout childhood. Even before we consciously know what a story is, we are collecting material for the 'self-defining story we will someday compose' (McAdams, 1997, p. 13). However, the development of a personal narrative is dependent on the ability to think abstractly, a cognitive achievement attained during adolescence. Accordingly, it is from late adolescence onwards that we begin to use the material and tools acquired thus far to form our life experiences into a coherent, purposeful and meaningful story. Through the adult years, we continually refashion our story in an effort to 'articulate a meaningful niche in the psychosocial world' and to provide our life with unity or purpose (McAdams, 1997, p. 5). Three of the seven key narrative elements identified by McAdams emerge during infancy and childhood, the fourth towards the end of adolescence and the remaining three during the years of adulthood.

Thus, for McAdams, personal identity in the modern world is a life story: 'If you want to know me, then you must know my story, for my story defines who I am. If *I* want to know *myself*, to gain insight into the meaning of my own life, then I, too, must come to know my own story' (McAdams, 1997, p. 11). Your work as occupational therapists will inevitably lead you to become involved in the discovery, creation and telling of clients' stories. It may also fall to you to be part of your clients' narratives as they incorporate into their life stories the nature and impact of whatever interaction you have with them.

The function of narrative

Narratives can help fulfil a number of psychological functions, such as preserving self-esteem or allocating responsibility elsewhere (Viney & Bousfield, 1991). Our role as active agent in the telling of our stories can be empowering (Viney, 1993). Think about Helen in our case study. At the moment she is floundering: tired, tearful, confused and not wanting to talk about her situation. It may be helpful in understanding Helen to see her as someone whose personal life story has lost its coherence and meaning and who, as yet, has not found a way to put it back together again. At present she does not feel as if she is an active agent in her own life story. Her family, on the other hand, are telling (if only to themselves) in a myriad of ways, different versions of her story. Helen will need to find her own voice in order to redefine for herself her post-CVA identity and gain some sense of control over her life.

We hear as well as tell stories about who we are. The stories that we hear in our family, school and immediate community (that is in what were described in Chapter 1 as our microsystems and interacting settings) teach us our place in the world, and give our lives some order and predictability. Narratives help us normalize our experiences. Stories which mirror our own lives reassure us that our experiences are normal, both in the sense of being understandable and in the sense of being shared by others. These stories will frequently reflect the 'social clock' of our society and form the basis of our assessments of what we 'should' be doing, and when. We evaluate ourselves either positively or negatively in relation to the events and timing of the social clock. The significance of age norms and the timing of life events has been a theme running through much of our consideration of the life course. It is important for you to remember that the life course of many of your clients will not mirror society's norms, and helping them to create an acceptable narrative may be a difficult, but important, aspect of your work with them.

Although the narratives within our society can give guidance and direction to our lives, they may, however, be imperfect guides (Cochran, 1997). Like an individual's life structure (Levinson *et al.*, 1978; Levinson, 1986), cultural narratives may become out of date and no longer compatible with the prevailing conditions of life. 'Lifted from conditions of life to which they did apply, these narratives might be described as anachronistic, impoverished, or distorted' (Cochran, 1997, p. 137). The notion of career choice as typically involving a once-and-for-all decision and of career development as typically being a smooth, upward progression are examples of such outmoded narratives.

In addition, narratives may conflict such that, to use Cochran's phrase, we may 'be torn between two narratives' (p. 137). A Western narrative emphasizing self-fulfilment may conflict with an Eastern one that emphasizes family obligation, such that second-generation immigrants may feel they have to choose between isolation from their family and stultification of personal dreams. Similarly, several people in our case study seem to feel torn between their own needs and plans and their obligations to Helen.

Furthermore, there may be situations for which no adequate narratives exist. Perhaps this is part of Helen's dilemma. Having experienced her CVA at the relatively young age of 52 years, she may simply not know what narratives are available to her. It may be that you have clients in this situation. A condition that may be familiar to you from your professional experience may be a total unknown to clients. This is where support and self-help groups can be useful in providing role models and a place where new life stories can be explored and constructed (Kurtz, 1997; Norcross *et al.*, 2000). We are able to generate multiple storylines to accommodate and account for our experiences (McLeod, 1997), and any one account is likely to be only a provisional interpretation. Whilst many of us will have a core narrative (Spence, 1987; Gustafson, 1992), a central or singular theme that underpins the various stories we tell, and which we repeat in different relationships at different points across the life course, it is more like a suggestive hypothesis than a confirmed generalization. Viney and Bousfield (1991) liken the core narrative to a 'statement of best fit'. It is not the only statement that could be made, but it is one that is plausible. The core narrative may be resilient, but it is not inviolable.

McAdams developed his theory of life story development on the basis of data from a 'Life Story Interview' that covered a range of topics. Look at Learning Task 7.2, which summarizes and invites you to respond to McAdams' interview schedule. In composing your own responses to the questions in this interview schedule, or

Learning Task 7.2   Exploring your story

For this exercise, you can work privately, although McAdams (1997) recommends working with a 'sympathetic listener', ideally a friend who has not to date been significant in influencing your life. What follows is a list of questions that should lead to a reasonably comprehensive account of your personal narrative and generate information about each of the key story elements identified by McAdams. It is a major undertaking and you may need to be selective in which questions you address. If you are reading this book as part of your training in occupational therapy, the activity may form a focus for some personal reflection work, or possibly be the basis of a course assignment. Only the broad introductory questions are included. The questions are based on the interview schedule developed by McAdams for his research. It is likely that in undertaking this Learning Task you can draw on your responses to earlier tasks that focused on your own experience, for example those in Chapter 3 (Life Events), Chapter 4 (Transition and Loss) and Chapter 5 (Stress and its Management).

1. Life chapters

Begin this exploration by identifying 'chapters' in your life. The goal is not to give the 'whole story', merely a sense of the story's outline, a table of contents:

   Think of your life as if it were a book, with each part of your life comprising a different chapter. Of course, the book is still unfinished, but it probably already contains several interesting and well-defined chapters. Divide your life into its major chapters, say between two and eight in number, and briefly describe each one. Think of this as a general table of contents for your book. Give each chapter a name and describe its overall contents. Discuss briefly the transition from one chapter to the next.

2. Key events

Reflect on some specific episodes in your past that stand out for some reason and are set in a particular time and place. Examples of key events could be:

- *A peak experience:* a high point in your life story.
- *A nadir experience:* a low point in your life story.
- *A turning point:* an episode where you underwent a significant change in your understanding of yourself.
- *An important early memory:* any memory, either positive or negative, from your childhood that stands out today and that is complete with setting, scene, characters, feelings and thoughts.
- *An important adolescent memory:* any memory, again either positive or negative, from your teenage years that stands out today.
- *An important adult memory:* a memory, positive or negative, that stands out from age 21 onwards.

3. Significant people

Now focus up to *four* of the most important people in your life story and ask yourself:

- What kind of relationship did, or do, I have with this person?
- What has been their impact on my life story?

4. Future script

Having thought about past events and influences, now consider the future.

- What do I think will happen next in my life story?
- What is my dream for the future?

5. Stresses and problems

Now consider in detail one or two areas where you are currently experiencing at least one of the following:

- significant stress
- a major conflict
- a difficult problem or challenge that must be addressed.

6. Personal ideology

In this section think about your fundamental beliefs and values: your spiritual, political, and philosophical position.

7. Overall life theme

As a finale, look back over your entire life story to see whether you can identify a central theme, message or idea: a core narrative.

in listening to the responses of others, much can be learnt about the content of life stories. However, much can also be learnt from listening to the *form* (or type) of story that is told, and also the *style* (or way) of telling it.

Narrative forms

Narrative forms, or types, are general storylines that underlie the plot and tensions of particular stories (Frank, 1995). You have already been asked to construct a personal narrative, in that the lifeline you will have drawn as part of Learning Task 7.1 can be thought of as a visual representation of your life story. Gergen and Gergen (1988; Gergen, 1988) use this linear, graphical representation of the life course as a basis for classifying different types of narratives or 'story lines'. They distinguish three simple story lines: a *progressive* narrative, where things get progressively better over time, is represented by an upwardly sloping graph, a *regressive* narrative, where events become increasingly negative, is represented by a downwards slope and a *stability* narrative, where the story line is largely unchanging, by a flat, horizontal line. This distinction has been used, for example, in exploring the personal narratives of people with multiple sclerosis (Robinson, 1990).

Generally, these simple forms will be combined within any one life course to produce a more complex structure. It is unlikely that your lifeline was a straight, unbending line. It is far more probable to have undulated up and down, with the degree of change being indicated by the height and depth of the undulations, and the pace of change indicated by the angle of slope. If you compare your lifeline with those of others, you will doubtless be struck by the differences between them: each is in its own way unique.

Nonetheless, literary scholars have long suggested that there are only a limited number of story forms. One of the best-known distinctions is that proposed by Frye (1957), who distinguishes between the story forms of *comedy, romance, tragedy* and *irony* (or *satire*) (see Salmon, 1985; Gergen, 1988). A comedy is not necessarily funny, although humour may play a part. In a *comedy*, a challenge or threat is overcome to yield social harmony and a happy ending.

Clients who make light, possibly through the use of humour, of their condition and difficulties may be constructing this type of story. Whilst they may value the 'happy ending' that such a story strives for, it is important that they are not being encouraged to minimize or hide concerns and worries that they could benefit from expressing.

In a *romance*, the main character emerges victorious from a series of challenges and threats that are overcome by idealism, love and personal commitments. So, Alison, for example, could describe her life in terms of an escape from the constraints of her background. Listeners would be expected to be enthralled and admiring of such a protagonist. In a *tragedy*, personal flaws and shortcomings lead to the defeat or demise of the main character. Happiness and position in society are lost. In a *satire* (or *irony*), the main character is defeated by insurmountable hurdles and the hopelessness of the situation. Beyond hope, these narratives are the representations of unrealized expectations and dreams. Clients will frequently find themselves faced with a tragic or satirical narrative, or with some combination of them both.

It is well, in work with clients, to reflect on the form their narrative takes for it will indicate much about their world view. If their narrative is of failure and loss, for example, do they see this as 'their fault' in some way – the consequence of their personal flaws or inadequacies (that is as a tragedy) – or do they place the responsibility elsewhere – the consequence of the situation they are in (that is as a satire)? Such interpretations may lead to different emotional responses: depression and a low sense of self-worth, for example, in the case of a tragic world view, or anger, blame and resentment in the case of a satiric perspective.

Although Frye's (1957) distinction between different story forms can be insightful, its value as a practical tool to guide understanding and practice is hampered by the fact that our colloquial understanding of something as comic, romantic, tragic or ironic may not accord with Frye's rather particular definitions of these terms. There are, however, other distinctions between different story forms that are more directly relevant to the health and social care setting, and our attention now turns to one of these: Frank's (1995) distinction between restitution, chaos and quest narratives. He writes about 'narratives of illness', although, in an attempt to distance our focus from a specifically medical emphasis, we prefer to talk of 'narratives of distress'.

Narratives of distress

Illness, disability or other forms of distress frequently take over clients' lives such that they lose any sense of control over what is happening to them. This is exacerbated by treatments which pass this control on to others, notably members of the health and social care professions. Frank (1995) argues that, in order to recover their voice (and, thereby, their control), those who are ill need to become storytellers.

Using the concept of 'narrative type', Frank describes three types of illness narrative: *restitution, chaos* and *quest*: 'Restitution stories attempt to outdistance mortality by rendering illness transitory. Chaos stories are sucked into the undertow of illness and the disasters that attend it. Quest stories meet suffering head on; they accept illness and seek to use it' (Frank, 1995, p. 115).

- *Restitution narratives:* The most common type of narrative, restitution narratives, contain a storyline whereby the person moves from health to illness, and then back to health again. This storyline can be both helpful and harmful. For people who are ill, it can be helpful to hear stories of others and their return to health. It can be consoling, giving people hope and the belief that they will recover. Thus, it is to be hoped that Helen from our case study will come to see her as experience as, at least to some extent, a restitution narrative. Although the state of health to which she may return is unlikely to be exactly what it was, a restitution narrative instils a belief in the possibility of recovery. On the downside, however, restitution narratives tend to give control for the restitution of health to the medical practitioner, and reflect medicine's emphasis on diagnosis, treatment and cure. Also, whilst many people do, indeed, return to health, some do not, and the social imperative to do so that is part and parcel of restitution narratives denies some people's experience of illness and its lasting effects (Thomas-MacLean, 2004).
- *Chaos narratives:* In contrast to restitution narratives, chaos narratives lack clear, linear movement and contain little hope that life will ever get better. These stories are described by Frank (1995) as 'anti-narrative', and reveal a sense of vulnerability, futility and impotence. This is resonant of the 'self-doubt' stage of the transition cycle that was discussed in Chapter 4. In our case study, Helen's current narrative may take this form.

However, as with the transition cycle, narrative understandings can change. Thus, whilst Helen is currently experiencing her life as chaotic, and lacking in narrative coherence, with time and appropriate support this may be transformed into a more positive and constructive understanding of her situation.

Our society is often uncomfortable with chaos stories, making it all the more important that health and social care practitioners should allow clients space to express them and should work hard to hear them. To ignore these stories, or to push people through them towards restitution narratives, risks denying important elements of clients' experiences, and contradicts the notion of client-centred practice. Although most people would prefer to avoid stories of chaos, they must be uncovered in order to enhance understanding of the meaning of illness and distress to those experiencing it.

- *Quest narratives:* Frank's third type of narrative, the quest, shows how illness may be considered useful: the teller accepts the illness and believes that something has been gained from the experience. There is resonance here with the notion of post-traumatic growth discussed in Chapter 4. Whilst losses are mourned, the emphasis is on the gains. The majority of published accounts of illness follow this format. The illness was a 'challenge' and an impetus for change. As with the concept of post-traumatic growth, however, a note of caution is in order with regard to quest narratives. These are narratives that are good to hear about, speaking, as they do, of triumph over adversity. However, clients should not be pushed towards expressing this type of narrative unless it has a genuine resonance with their experience. Being told to 'look on the bright side', 'count their blessings' or remember how 'things could be a lot worse' may not be helpful to someone who is currently unable to see any positive side to their experience.

A quest narrative differs from a restitution narrative in that it represents change rather than recovery. Thomas-MacLean (2004) researched the stories of breast cancer sufferers, and discusses the quest narrative of one of her participants who framed her experience as 'a lesson learned':

Framing one's quest as a lesson may be a means of acknowledging that the experience of illness is involuntary, but that the meaning one creates from illness experiences is somewhat voluntary. The implication of framing one's narrative as a lesson is indicative of a blurring of the boundaries between illness and meaning, as lessons do not imply active choice to change, but a response to external force. (Thomas-MacLean, 2004, p. 1654)

Whilst quest stories can be seen as therapeutic, there is a risk that they present storylines that are 'too clean', resolutions that are 'too complete' and implicitly deprecate those who 'fail to rise out of their own ashes' (Frank, 1995, p. 135). Such failure contradicts the cultural imperative or social prescription for tidy, or wrapped-up, narratives, which creates the assumption that we can and should 'put the past behind us', and that once treatments have ended the illness is no longer worthy of discussion. Again, awareness of and attention to chaos narratives reminds us to be cautious about accepting quest narratives. However, it may also be that clients offer quest narrative as a defensive mechanism that enables them to avoid confronting the full implications of their condition. Telling a quest narrative may be their coping mechanism, and health and social care professionals need to be hesitant of taking this option from them.

These different types of narrative can intermingle. Thus, chaos narratives are often contained within the other two story forms as, for example, when the possibility of the recurrence of an illness introduces chaotic elements into what was until then a restitution story. With chronic illnesses and permanent disabilities, restitution is not possible, and the realization of this may lead to what Frank terms narrative 'wreckage'. Out of this wreckage, a quest narrative may emerge: 'What is quested for may never be wholly clear, but the quest is defined by the ill person's belief that something is to be gained through the experience' (Frank, 1995, p. 115).

Story styles

Rather than focusing on the building blocks of the overall life narrative (as does McAdams) or the overarching story form (as do Frye and Frank), Janine Roberts (1994), a family therapist, looks at how particular stories within that narrative are told: how complete are they, how fluid are they and how do they relate to other stories the client tells? In total, she distinguishes six story styles: *intertwined, isolated, incomplete, unspoken, frozen* and *evolving*. Intertwined and isolated stories are distinguished by a concern with the amount and nature of resonance between different stories. With incomplete and silenced stories, the main issue is about gaps: why and how they occurred, whether they can be filled and the implications of so doing. With frozen and evolving stories, the focus is on movement and change versus stagnation and fixity.

- *Intertwined stories:* Intertwined stories resonate, either because of their similarities or because of their differences, with stories of another time and/or place. This can be a wonderful resource. Through such resonance, we can use the stories we have already lived and heard to understand our present and decide how to act. However, stories may become enmeshed, or possibly soldered together, rather than merely intertwined. When stories are too richly cross-joined, the first story seems to overwhelm the second story with interpretations of behaviour and actions and with its own emotional field. People involved in the second story then find few possibilities of coming to their own meaning-making of the events in their lives. The meaning has already been passed from the first story (Roberts, 1994, p. 14). A task for therapist and client is to unravel this tangled web so that each story can stand on its own, with its uniqueness and integrity respected.
- *Isolated stories:* Just as stories can become overly intertwined, so too may they be overly isolated. If we are blind to the ways in which our stories are linked, we cannot learn from our experience. Instead, we are forever reinventing the wheel, as it were. Exploring the ways in which stories from different life stages or from different areas of our life may be linked can help give us access to different levels of meaning and interpretation of our lives. It is the antithesis of the extreme compartmentalization of our lives into categories such work/play, home/school or now/then.
- *Incomplete stories:* Through a range of disruptions – changing school or job, geographic moves, family break-ups – we may lose contact with our stability zones: the 'locations, symbols, people, and activities' (Roberts, 1994, p. 16) that may otherwise inhabit

our stories. In the upheaval of moving house, photos, letters and other memorabilia may be thrown out or lost. Family rituals and reunions, whilst they may constrain and confine us, also help us know who we are. When parents divorce, children may lose contact with one set of grandparents, thereby losing access to a range of stories about the family. Stories are patchy (McLeod, 1997) or incomplete, with crucial episodes missing, stages skipped and causal links omitted.

- *Unspoken stories:* Unspoken stories are perhaps the most difficult and potentially risky stories to work with. Whereas the gaps in incomplete stories can be openly acknowledged and addressed, stories that have been silenced or are secret present complex issues of safety and disclosure: 'When there are secret stories in a family, people live with a subterranean text. Meaning is unclear, and there are often hidden alliances and coalition' (Roberts, 1994, p. 18). Clients may be fearful of expressing some of their concerns, and therapists must listen and pay attention to the unspoken: 'it is the continuous backdrop for that which can be told' (p. 9).

- *Frozen stories:* Frozen stories are told repeatedly in the same way. They are static, rigid and unbending. Their content and assumed meaning is so familiar and unquestioned that we may be blink-ered to alternative stances; it is as if there were only one way of telling the story, and, indeed, only one story to tell. 'But that's the way it is,' we may say to ourselves, 'it always has been, and always will be.' A role for therapists is to help clients liberate themselves from the constraints of such frozen or rigidly told stories, melting the ice, one could say.

- *Evolving stories:* From a life course perspective, a role for health and social care professionals can be seen as the nurturance and encouragement of evolving stories. Not only do illness and other personal, family and cultural stories need to be told, but they need to be told (and heard) across time, enabling them to be understood on different levels. As we develop, we are able to make meaning in different ways cognitively, and draw on new knowledge and sets of life experiences to help us to interpret events (McAdams, 1997). Such stories represent quest narratives (Frank, 1995).

Having read through these descriptions of different story styles, turn now to Learning Task 7.3.

Learning Task 7.3 Exploring story styles

Turn back to the case study account in Chapter 0 and read through it again, keeping in mind as you do so the different story styles identified by Roberts (1994). Try to identify these different styles in the stories of the various characters. Also, think about clients you work with: what story styles are they using?

- *Intertwined stories:* Look for examples of learning and meaning being transferred from one story to another. Try to find examples where this is helpful, and examples where it is a hindrance.
- *Isolated stories:* Try to identify instances where links and resonances between different stories are missed. What could be the consequences of making these connections explicit?
- *Incomplete stories:* What gaps are there in the stories? Is it important to fill these gaps? Can they be filled, or is the information lost for ever?
- *Unspoken stories:* Are there any stories that have been silenced? Does it seem that there are things that cannot be talked about? Does this matter? What might happen were the stories to be told in full?
- *Frozen stories:* Are there stories that are told repeatedly in the same way? Why do you think the story takes the form it does? What would be the implications of changing the story?
- *Evolving stories:* Try to find examples of stories that have evolved over time. What supported and helped these stories to evolve? Are they continuing to develop? What may encourage or hinder this?

The use of metaphor

At various points in this work book, we have used a number of everyday phrases and analogies to convey what we meant. This mirrors much human interaction, including that between clients and the people who work with them. It is not only the overall shape, tone or style of a client's story that is relevant. Attention to the words and phrases they use can reveal much about how they view and experience their world (Bury, 2001). Sensitivity to clients' feelings and mood is crucial, and very often you will find that these are not expressed directly. Rather than saying 'I am feeling sad, worried, anxious, hopeful etc.', clients will often indicate their emotions indirectly through the use of metaphor. Clients will also use metaphor to circumscribe and frame possible solutions to the problem areas in their lives (Mallinson *et al.*, 1996). Being attuned to this, and developing your own appreciation of and capacity to use metaphor, can be a valuable professional skill. Learning Task 7.4 helps you to explore this issue further.

Learning Task 7.4   Metaphors and mood

The aim of this task is to increase your awareness of and sensitivity to the indirect expression of feelings and mood through the use of metaphors.

- Begin by identifying some the metaphorical expressions or feelings that have been used in this work book. You will find Chapter 4 to be a particularly well-populated hunting ground. Being 'frozen in our tracks' was the first one we used in that chapter. Note down in your Learning Journal all the others that you can find, linking these phrases to the sequential stages of the transition cycle.
- Now add to your list by thinking about others phrases that might have been used. Include phrases you have heard clients use or, indeed, you yourself have used.
- During the next few days, as you go about your daily life, listen out for metaphors that clients, friends, family, characters in books and people on the radio or TV use to describe their feelings and emotional state when talking about significant life events.

Note down these phrases as a way of expanding your vocabulary for describing, and for becoming attuned to, feelings and other psychological states.

Conclusion

Wicks and Whiteford (2003) identify four significant reasons life stories are important to occupational therapists:

- First, the philosophical foundations of a narrative approach are compatible with the humanist values and assumptions of occupational therapy: 'The use of life stories preserves the integrity of individuals, accepts individuals' experiences as credible, and recognises that individuals interact within a variety of contexts over time' (p. 87).

- Second, there is a strong connection between stories and occupation, in that stories are accounts of people's occupations, and it is through stories that people give meaning to their occupational experiences. Life stories are particularly useful and relevant because they can provide rich information about the range and form of occupations in which people participate. Life stories can also augment understandings about the meaning, experience and function of occupation throughout a person's life course.
- Third, since life stories are set within contexts of time and place, they provide a contextual framework within which to understand a person's occupational experiences.
- Fourth, the sharing of life stories can yield many personal benefits, including a clearer perspective on personal experiences and feelings; improved self-knowledge, self-image and self-esteem; satisfaction and pleasure from sharing one's own story; opportunity to release or purge certain burdens, and validate personal experience; and the acquisition of a sense of community.

By forming narratives, we order our experiences in a way that expresses (or, perhaps, creates) a sense of ourselves as intentional agents (Lynch, 1997). It is a way of attaining some sense of personal control. 'If we do not exactly write the plots of our lives, nevertheless it is we alone who create our own stories. Agency lies not in governing what shall happen to us, but in creating what we make of what happens. We ourselves construct the meaning of our story' (Salmon, 1985, pp. 138–9). Helping clients to incorporate experiences into a meaningful life story is important in developing their sense of identity and self-worth. It is also something that occupational therapists, and other health and social care practitioners, should do for themselves in relation to their own life stories. The remaining two chapters of this work book aim to facilitate this by placing the occupational therapist centre stage. Chapter 8 explores the 'career stories' that occupational therapists do or may tell about their working life and Chapter 9 focuses on the topics of continuing professional development and the therapeutic use of self.

8. *Becoming and Belonging as an Occupational Therapist*

This chapter explores the ways in which life course theory underpins the career path of occupational therapists. It is presented rather differently from other chapters in that it is not based on our case study (p. 6) but on the career stories of real occupational therapists who participated in a study about occupational therapy career pathway experience (Wright, 2007). The chapter includes quotations and career histories from a number of research participants, and we wish to thank them for making this possible. All names have, of course, been changed, along with any other details that could identify them. As usual, there are Learning Tasks asking you to reflect on your own experience and to think about how these real-life experiences fit with theory.

All of the people who have offered their stories here have worked in practice and then moved into occupational therapy education. In doing this, they have first developed expertise and mastery as practitioners, and then made a move within the profession to a setting where they were novices. This is the extreme case of that which we all experience when we move away from one area of work, or from one employer, to another. All of the participants are or have been senior practitioners, and their stories illustrate the twists and turns of a career journey, in particular illustrating the power of professional socialization. We hope that by looking at the careers and issues of others you will be able to gain some insight into your own pathways, both those already trodden and those still to be experienced.

To set the scene, we are starting with an overview of one career story, that of Harjit. Her story shows how a career path is the outcome of many factors: interest, ambition, family demands and circumstances, opportunity and chance, to name just a few.

Career Story: Harjit

Harjit was the second of three children in a Sikh family. They lived in the town where Harjit and her brothers had been born and where her father, a businessman, had also been born. Her family formed an important part of Harjit's life as much time was spent with relatives. Harjit's mother had been born in India, coming over from Amritsar at age 19 to marry Kannan, Harjit's father. Harjit wore Western clothes and the family were quite Westernized. The one exception to this was that Harjit's parents assumed they would choose her marriage partner. Harjit was happy about this, confident that her parents would make a good choice with her best interests at heart. She wanted to go to university to study occupational therapy, and marry after this. Her parents were in agreement with this and Harjit went to university 50 miles from her home town. She enjoyed her course and her student life. During the third year of her course, she became engaged to a distant cousin and found planning and arranging the wedding thoroughly enjoyable and very absorbing. She and her husband married soon after Harjit's graduation and subsequently went to live with his parents in a city a 100 miles south of where she had been born. She and her new husband got on very well and the marriage was successful from the start. Her mother-in-law, however, was surprised to find that Harjit wanted to find a job rather than start a family. Harjit was determined though and, supported by her husband, she obtained a rotational post at the local acute trust. Harjit enjoyed the work very much; she enjoyed the purpose of working with the clients and the occupational therapy community she worked with. She became particularly interested in the developing area of accident and emergency work and worked hard as she gained seniority to get an accident and emergency service piloted and then established in the trust. Harjit's husband was fully supportive and proud of Harjit's tenacity. He too was very determined to develop his own career as an accountant, and they were able to find much in common to strengthen their relationship in their mutual ambition in their own careers. By this time, they had been married for five years and had moved into a house of their own near to Harjit's in-laws. Because of her passion for her profession and her interest in her particular area of work, Harjit began to become involved with the College of Occupational Therapy. This meant a certain amount of travelling to and from London. Harjit was happy and fulfilled, and her parents and in-laws, although slightly at a loss, were happy for her. She took continuing professional development seriously, and completed a master's degree in occupational therapy, studying part-time whilst still working full-time After seven years of marriage, Harjit became pregnant and had a baby girl. Delighted as she was with her daughter, she was keen to return to work to take up a part-time post as head occupational therapist managing a service that included accident and emergency as well as orthopaedics, neurology and general medicine. With the full support of her husband, Harjit returned to work when her daughter was eight months old. Harjit's sister-in-law looked after the new baby while Harjit worked 18 hours a week. Although Harjit's job was important to her, she was surprised to find that she was much less energetic at work and less single-minded than she had been, her real interest now being her daughter. Nonetheless, she continued in the same job until another daughter was born four years later. This time Harjit took a full year of maternity leave before returning to work. When she had been back at work for a few months, Harjit began to realize that she was bored in her current job and needed a change of direction in her career. This presented difficulties, as she did not want to leave occupational therapy, or the area in which she had specialized and developed expertise. She would have been prepared to drop down a grade to take up a new career pathway, although she was unclear as to what it might be. Important as her relationships at work were to her, they had become somewhat eclipsed by her involvement with her immediate and extended family. An advertisement for a post as an occupational therapy lecturer at a local university caught her eye. She applied and was offered the post.

Spend some time reflecting on Harjit's career to date. Learning Task 8.1 suggests some particular issues to consider.

Learning Task 8.1   Reflections on Harjit's career

Before focusing on the specific questions below, jot down in your Learning Journal your immediate responses to Harjit's story. Then, consider her experience: what do you think the key issues were for her?

• Can you identify with any of the issues Harjit faced, either in her career or in her life as a whole?

- Do you think she made wise decisions? With the information available, do you think you would have chosen differently?
- Reading through Harjit's career story, what factors do you think contributed to her success? Think about factors within Harjit herself and factors within her environment, particularly her social and familial network. Do you think you could offer her some suggestions for making her life either easier or more fulfilled?
- Although Harjit switched to part-time employment after the birth of her first daughter, she and her husband remained a dual-career couple. How do you feel about this? Supposing Harjit had been the accountant, and her husband the occupational therapist, how do you think they might have managed the career–family balance then? What would you have done?

Becoming and belonging

The underpinning professional enterprise for all occupational therapists is to develop professional skills and to become and belong as an occupational therapist. The work of Wenger (1999, 2003), Skovholt and Ronnestad (1995) and Levinson (1990) provides central frameworks and concepts for understanding these processes. 'Becoming' speaks of growth and development, of changing rather than remaining static and of gaining expertise and confidence. 'Belonging' here means feeling part of a group, of having a sense of a shared identity, which gives rise to a shared community. The need to belong to a group is felt deeply by almost all people, and this need extends to the professional arena (Wenger, 1999). However, during the course of any occupational therapy career, moves are made – from workplace to workplace, from role to role. Change is also imposed on the work milieu and practice from outside.

The enormity of the endeavour of leaving a place of belonging and moving to another where the whole work of becoming and then belonging has to begin again is always hard work. The therapists sharing their stories here described this transition, many of them very movingly. We can see this in terms of the 'expert to novice' transition. Even if you are still at the threshold of your occupational therapy career, you will still have experienced the process of becoming, belonging and leaving a situation, group or community. Learning Task 8.2 is designed to help you reflect on this.

Learning Task 8.2   Becoming, belonging . . . and leaving

Try to identify from your own experience situations where you chose or were forced to move on from people, places or roles that had, over a long period, become familiar and taken-for-granted elements of your day-to-day life. Leaving primary school at age 11 could be one example. Leaving school to go to university, or moving with your family either to a different part of the country or to another country altogether, could be other possibilities. This may be the moment to refer back to the personal life space you depicted in Learning Task 2.1 (p. 39), the stability zone activity found in Learning Task 2.2 (p. 46) or the transitions you identified in Learning Task 4.2 (p. 81).

- How did these endings feel? What were the positives? What was difficult? Did you find strategies that worked? When (if at all) did you feel at home in the new situation? Had you 'become'? Did you 'belong'?

Those of you who complete this task will doubtless be at different stages in your occupational therapy career. Some of you will still be students – still at the 'becoming' stage with regard to your profes-sional identity. But all of you can think back to when you decided to study occupational therapy.

- When did you decide to study occupational therapy? What were the reasons for your choice? Who or what influenced you? To what extent has occupational therapy turned out to be what you expected it to be? What has surprised you about it? How have all these issues affected your professional identity as an occupational therapist?

In undertaking your journey to becoming an occupational thera-pist in a way that is internalized for you personally there are many challenges and much learning to address. At each change, to a greater or lesser extent, you leave behind a community of practice which you know well, in which you might have been well sup-ported and for which you had been well prepared, and enter into something new. The occupational therapist moving into an educa-tional setting is perhaps the most extreme example of 'in-career change'. Leaving clinical care (whether for education or other roles, such as management) requires both confidence and courage, something that we suggest is often not articulated or even actively considered by those who take this step. This means that people are likely to be relatively unprepared to confront some aspects of the personal journey involved in these career moves. One occupational therapist said about the move into occupational therapy education, 'I thought I'd be working with OTs.' She went on to say that she had been disappointed and, indeed, wrong-footed by the fact that 'it wasn't like that at all'.

In entering the world of occupational therapy education, the work being taken on involves preparing others for a community to which the occupational therapists making this transition no longer wholly belong themselves. At the very least they have left the community of practitioners for a time, and for some they have actively rejected it. How can these colleagues find a community of practice to belong to? Who and what are they to become?

One woman, Karen, expressed the desire for becoming and belonging when no longer engaged in practice when she said, 'I want to know what I am and others to know, to be able to articulate it.' She further reflected on what becoming and belonging meant for her and explained that part of her reason for coming into occupational therapy education was, 'I want to develop fully as a professional.' Karen clearly felt that the academic and education area of occupational therapy was a legitimate part of the profession which would add depth to her professional self. She added, 'I want to be what I am professionally. My work is part of me.' In this way, Karen indicates that professional becoming and belonging is located in a much more complete sense of personal becoming. There is a clear sense that Karen is driven by the belief that occupational therapy is not just a profession, still less a job, but a central part of her identity. This is a clear example of 'ideas and values' operating as a significant stability zone.

This desire to *be* in some sense what one *does* amongst the community of occupational therapists does not fade because the arena of professional life has changed. Something that is clear is that professional identity is maintained at its best and most compelling within a group (Skovholt & Ronnestad, 1995; Wenger, 1999, 2003). The need to belong in a professional sense, for support and development, is well rehearsed; indeed, one occupational therapist expressed this unambiguously when, describing her professional development needs, she said, 'I want to belong to a group.'

A sense of belonging is a human essential, and when the profession is closely integrated into the sense of self, a professional group assumes great significance. Within the study into the career pathways of occupational therapists, there was much that underscored the need to maintain a sense of becoming and belonging within whatever community one was working in. There seemed to be two strands to this. One strand, which the people who participated in the research project articulated very clearly, was the sense of belonging and continuing to belong as an occupational therapist even if they no longer actually worked clinically (or, indeed, worked as an occupational therapist at all). In fact, an expert academic, who was perfectly comfortable in her academic role, said quite clearly: 'I *really* am an OT.' In saying this, she was not undermining herself in her current role but simply stating where her deepest allegiances and sense of belonging lay.

There was another strand underlying this sense of belonging: a sense of becoming in terms of 'growing up'. Various expressions of this were given by the research project participants. One woman, Gemma, explained: 'I work with OTs. I know what they're about, what OT is about, what it should be. I've grown up in it.' Speaking of how she felt about herself when she moved from clinical practice to occupational therapy education, she said: 'I won't let that sense of what I am go.'

Gemma shows us here her need to have a community to be a part of and her determination to preserve her feeling of belonging to it. But she also shows something else in speaking of her 'sense of what I am'. Her belonging is profoundly internalized. She feels that to lose her sense of belonging to this community would be to become less herself, to lose something vital and profound about who she is. Many of the research participants noted the philosophical fit between themselves and the philosophical purposes of occupational therapy. One participant, who had been in education for many years explained: 'The actual basics of OT, the philosophy behind it, fits me, and I can use it. I can be an OT anywhere.' Reflecting on this, she added: 'I can't imagine why anyone does anything else really.' It would be valuable to pause here for a while, and reflect on what being an occupational therapist means to you. Turn to Learning Task 8.3 if you would like some structure to guide your thoughts.

Learning Task 8.3   Being an occupational therapist

Your sense of what it means to you to be an occupational therapist
will change and develop over the course of your career. Reflect on this
using the following prompts.

When you applied to study occupational therapy, you probably had
to explain and justify your decision, on paper and/or in a face-to-face
interview. Think about, and note down in your Learning Journal,
what you said then.

Look back to the final section of Learning Task 8.2 and remind
yourself of the comments you made about the reasons for and influences on your career choice.

Now think more about your professional identity as it is now.

- How do you feel about being an occupational therapist?
- What does it mean to you?
- Is it part of your sense of self?
- To what extent do you share its philosophical values?

There is, within the occupational therapy family, the definite idea
that alongside a sense of belonging there is also a sense of becoming.
'I knew where I started from and where I'd got to,' said another
research participant. She seems to be referring here to her journey
as an occupational therapist from novice to expert. Whilst, ideally,
the personal fit is significant, being an occupational therapist is not
simply about valuing the philosophy. It is also about having mastery
of skills and having tools for practice. There is a journey to make
and work to do in acquiring these, and during the acquisition and
professional development the person is changed in terms of their
professional outlook and their professional needs (Skovholt &
Ronnestad, 1995; Wenger, 1999). The belonging is to a community
of practice (Wenger, 1999, 2003) and to a professional identity
(Skovholt & Ronnestad, 1995; Skovholt, 2001), and it is very
important.

As expertise develops, so the sense of confidence grows, until it
is strong enough to be maintained even when away from a concen-
trated group of occupational therapy colleagues. One person, talking
about being an occupational therapist in a multidisciplinary service,
felt that at this particular stage her confidence and expertise were
such that the dialogue with others in fact supported her own profes-

sional identity. She said about her work at that time: 'You'd think then that, as it was more collaborative, you'd have more overlap and less professional identity. But in reality, because we talked more, we were happy about each other's roles and I think that gave us [the occupational therapists] a stronger professional identity.' What this quotations seems to imply is that this occupational therapist's sense of confidence and expertise was not maintained by isolation from challenge but rather by an ability to work with others and still know her own role and value, and to know what she actually had to offer.

Of course, it is possible to belong to more than one group – indeed, we all do so, at least once we have passed infancy. It is also possible to grow out of one group and into another. We usually do. One research participant reflected something of this when she said in her interview: 'Actually, I think I've grown past it. It isn't me any more, or not all of me, in work terms. But in personal ways I have become an OT. I can't change that; I don't want to.' The speaker here offers a complex and subtle reflection on her career path: she says that she no longer wishes to *practise* occupational therapy, in her case in the NHS, but she does not say that she does not want to *be* an occupational therapist. Indeed, she suggests that this would be neither possible nor desirable. Nonetheless, she no longer wishes to function as a clinical practitioner, saying, interestingly, that she has grown out of it. She suggested that she wanted to take up a new challenge and so sought a new environment and direction. She did not, or could not, perhaps, contemplate changing what she was: an occupational therapist. In this personal sense, she belonged irrevocably to the community of occupational therapists, whilst hinting that she may also belong elsewhere and perhaps become something else as well. There are choices and opportunities ahead.

This chapter opened with the career narrative of an occupational therapist who, after many years' experience as a practitioner, was about to embark on a new, albeit connected, career as an occupational therapy educator. The chapter finishes with another career narrative, this time provided by an experienced academic, who we will call Jeanette. Her story focuses on the theme of changed identity during her career journey, enabling us to learn much from it. Jeanette expresses many of the themes which had emerged from the stories of other participants in the research. It has an extra dimension in that it tells a story which had a comfortable end point for this participant, where becoming and belonging has occurred (at least for now), and which is clearly seen as part of a personal journey. As you read through the coming section, try to make links between what Jeanette is saying and feeling and the theoretical concepts you have encountered in the book. Also reflect on whether there are comparisons with your own experiences.

Career Story: Jeanette

Jeanette began by saying that her move into academia had been made partly because of her personal domestic circumstances and partly because she was at a point in her life and career where she was seeking a new challenge and direction. In this, of course, she was similar to Harjit. Having reached an expert level in her clinical work, Jeanette had begun to feel frustrated by the constraints of the NHS, and she felt the need to develop further. The opportunity to take up a post in occupational therapy education came up and she made the move. She went on to say:

> My intention had been to move back into a clinical post after five years, but this didn't work out, for two reasons. One reason was that I wanted to be involved in pioneering degree education in occupational therapy. The second reason was that my original intention was rather naive. I had thought that five years would be sufficient time to become a competent educator, but this wasn't in fact true. Five years in education means that an individual only sees one cohort of students start and complete their training programme. In reality, I was only just beginning to have an influence on designing the curriculum that reflected the changes that were occurring not only in practice but also those that were occurring in pedagogy, or probably more accurately in androgogy.

One thing that is quite clear here is that the new work role met a need for Jeanette. She was enjoying the challenges and opportunities offered to her. This is not to be underestimated in terms of people's motivation towards making successful change (Goodman *et al.*, 2006; Pedler *et al.*, 2006). Timing is also an issue here. In higher education, timescales are often much longer than they are in clinical practice. Client care is relatively immediate and it required considerable refocusing for Jeanette to adjust to the much longer gestation period in occupational therapy education. The same is true of working in management, and this is something to remember when seeking to negotiate a career change. For those who go into occupational therapy education, the length of student programmes lends a degree of stability and longevity to the life of an academic, something which is generally lacking in the arena of health and social care. Jeanette now recognizes this; she knows the culture and rhythms of higher education and can make calculations about how to be involved, and about how to pursue what is important to her. Jeanette's experience shows how drawn out the process of becoming can be. We need time to make a change and to join a new community, and this shows in this particular narrative. Jeanette's identity as an occupational therapy educator, her orientation towards education and her views on the development of the occupational therapy profession emerged and developed over a period of some five years. For people moving from clinical practice to management, it may similarly be expected to take a number of years before they feel truly at home in the new role.

For Jeanette, it is not that she has moved away from considering herself an occupational therapist. Indeed, she still declares her intention to return to practice, believing that this is her true profession and career path. However, as she herself acknowledged, she was not actually all that serious about seeking to make this return to clinical practice happen. She reflected that she felt reluctant to admit to herself, and to others, that she no longer wanted to return to clinical practice. Not only was she enjoying her new work but she was beginning to feel very energized by it. She said:

> This was a stimulating and dynamic time to be involved in OT education. So the time wasn't right for me to move back into a clinical post.

We can see Jeanette at this point as having reached a stage on the way to belonging to a new community. She expresses the desire to be part of it, and the confidence to feel that she has a contribution to make. There is a sense of personal power and of the ability to influence. Interestingly the area of influence is specifically occupational therapy education, and so the stages of becoming are negotiated by maintaining old areas of stability (Pedler *et al.*, 2006) as part of the strategy for making the change more easily.

Jeanette became engaged in research, and again found this stimulating. This helped her to maintain her interest in the opportunities of her current post:

> which left me with the desire to be involved in further research.

Research has significant status in academic life (Henkel, 2000), and beginning to participate in this may be seen as another stage of becoming for Jeanette, giving her confidence and placing her on another part of the academic trajectory. The opportunities offered by new roles, and the value that we attach to them, make a great difference to how we feel about the changes we make.

Clearly defined roles can offer markers on the road to becoming, and in Jeanette's narrative a particular and senior role is cited as important. Already an expert educator, Jeanette is still undertaking the journey along the academic career path. She is typically modest about her achievement but recognizes its significance:

> The post of head of the department of occupational therapy was advertised, and I was encouraged to apply. And surprisingly, I was offered the post. This was a significant milestone in my career.

Jeanette's new role was specific and well defined, giving a clear purpose to her work. She saw her personal endeavour as making occupational therapy and occupational therapy educators accepted and respected within higher education. Feeling that occupational therapy did not have a high status in higher education, Jeanette was determined to change this perception. This indicates considerable confidence – the confidence of someone who has expertise (Benner, 1989) as well as firmness of purpose.

> It soon became evident to me as a manager and head of department that if we, as occupational therapy lecturers, wished to be accepted legitimately as academics we would need to be actively involved in research. In addition, we would require staff with doctoral qualifications.

Here we see that a part of Jeanette's new stage of becoming implies that she has a sense of possible belonging and of what it would take to belong. She also wished to bring her community of occupational therapy educators with her. Henkel (2000) would agree that this emphasis on research and, in particular, on recognized and measurable success in the area was entirely appropriate in a university setting This is not often the case in practice settings, and it is vital to understand what is valued in whatever community we find ourselves working in. If we are going to fit into our community of practice, we need to engage with its concerns and values. If we cannot share its values and priorities, it might be the wrong community for us.

Jeanette's narrative is a success story, and illustrates the pathway of someone who, over time, successfully integrated her professional identities and slowly, by means of step changes, came to belong to the academic community and yet maintain a core identity within the occupational therapy family. She also developed an expertise in her new arena of practice: she has negotiated the journey from expert to novice and to expert again. One thing that has emerged from both the research data and the literature (Wenger, 1999, 2003; Skovholt, 2001) is that once an area of expertise is established then confidence is gained to look at other areas. In the same vein, a novice whose whole attention is of necessity attuned to gaining core practice skills is unlikely to be able to attend to issues beyond this immediate concern. Moving along the pathway to expertise (Benner, 1989) – or, to reframe the notion, to move through becoming to belonging (Wenger, 1999) – allows the practitioner to develop new areas of interest. We need to be aware of where we are in our own progression so that we can have the appropriate expectations of ourselves and decide which change management strategies will help us most in our transition. We also need to be aware that we will have to reflect on changes in the emphases within our professional identities. Jeanette clearly demonstrates this:

I had become more actively interested in strategies for teaching students. So, on reflection, I could see that this was actually quite a key time, and I began to question whether I was an occupational therapist with an interest in education or whether I was an educator in occupational therapy.

In her statement, Jeanette describes the move away from 'occupational therapist' practice as her most significant professional identity. At the time it happened she did not notice the change. It was only on reflection that it was identified as 'a key time'. It is well attested (Schon, 1995) that reflection is a valuable tool in practice and development, both in moving from novice to expert and in the process of becoming and belonging. Jeanette's experience illustrates this, and ties in with her developing interests around a new endeavour. Nonetheless, the underpinning of occupational therapy in some form is apparent and maintained.

Jeanette's narrative illustrates and speaks eloquently of the process of becoming. The belonging in this case also implies a letting-go of supportive structures and a confirming community with a single identity. In the process, some stability zones will be lost. Instead, there is more dependence on a personal sense of the endeavour itself. This is something we must all expect as we move through our occupational therapy career paths.

There is something about articulating the new role that is like learning a language: practice in articulating gives confidence and meaning, and this, in turn, helps in the establishment of the new role and identity (Goffman, 1959). We hope that it will help all of us who look at this book to understand and manage our careers better as they progress and present us with opportunities and dilemmas. With this in mind, the final chapter of this work book focuses, like the present one, on the occupational therapist. On this occasion, whilst it makes reference to the career story of another occupational therapist, it is mainly concerned with your own professional development.

The present chapter ends with another Learning Task, this time one that asks you to think about and imagine your future. It addresses the question of what you will do to ensure that you both 'become' and 'belong' in your professional life. Find time to consider Learning Task 8.4.

Learning Task 8.4   Somewhere over the rainbow?

Reflect on your current career aspirations. What will you become? Where will you belong?

Take a little time to think about where you are now on your career path, where you have come from and where you wish to move to. Reflect on your current expectations of yourself: are they manageable, realistic, too modest? What strategies could move you towards your goals? What other goals do you have outside as well as inside your career? What alternatives could you consider?

(We suggest that you use the technique of force-field analysis, introduced in Learning Task 6.2 (p. 120), as a framework for considering these questions.)

9. *Developing Professional Practice*

Many of the Learning Tasks in this work book ask you in one way or another to think about your own life course experience. The rationale for this is based on the belief, first, that the life course concepts considered are as relevant to your life as they are to the lives of your clients and, second, that our life course experiences, and what we make of them, are key resources that we bring to and call on in our work with clients. This chapter advances this line of thinking by focusing explicitly on aspects of the person of the therapist, and notably in terms of the therapeutic use of self and in relation to the issue of continuing professional development.

As with the previous chapter, we set the scene with another career story of an occupational therapist: Ian. His story demonstrates some of the challenges of developing a career, and the very important role of personal motivations and goals in defining what we mean by 'career success and satisfaction'.

Career Story: Ian

Ian had been a teacher of craft design and technology for 20 years. He had begun to find teaching more and more of a strain, and was increasingly disillusioned by it. He was single, but had a close circle of friends and an extended family to which he was very close. He was neither lonely nor discontented with his life in terms of relationships. He was a keen gardener, and had an allotment which took up time and provided part of his social life. A cousin of his was an occupational therapist and after some time talking things over with her and visiting her at work he decided to apply for an accelerated programme for graduates to train as occupational therapists.

Ian found the course very tiring and challenging, but also exciting and absorbing. He was convinced that this was the right choice for him, although he did find it difficult to move from a teaching perspective to an enabling one. Despite this, he felt that on the whole he was able to derive more help than hindrance from his previous professional experience. He was particularly interested in working with those with learning disabilities. On graduation, Ian obtained a post with social services, and some of his clients had learning disabilities. He developed this part of his work with enthusiasm and joined the College of Occupational Therapists' specialist section for those working in the learning disability field.

A post came up for an occupational therapist to work at a college for young people (18–25 years) with learning disabilities. The post was to be particularly focused on the development of independent living skills. Ian applied for the post with great enthusiasm, and was very disappointed when it was offered to someone else. He then applied unsuccessfully for two more posts which were specifically concerned with learning disabled clients. Feedback from his interviews was largely positive: it had not been that Ian lacked the qualities or experience they were looking for, simply that other applicants had been even stronger. One of these posts would have involved moving to the other end of the country, and Ian admitted to feeling some relief that his life was not going to be turned upside down by such a major change and that he was not going to have to abandon the beloved allotment that he had spend so many years nurturing and developing. Nonetheless, he began to feel low and a little restless in his current job. He realized that he was a valued member of his present organization and began to wonder about promotion in his current post. However, it seemed unlikely to him that there would be any opportunities in the immediate future, and so he put the idea to one side.

During his annual appraisal meeting, Ian talked with his line manager about his unsuccessful job applications and his vague dissatisfaction with his present role. She had always had a high opinion of Ian's abilities and had been surprised that his job hunting had not been successful. Together, they started to explore whether they could try to reconfigure Ian's work role in order to both advance the work of the department and create a career development opportunity which was to his liking. They agreed that Ian would outline a proposal for developing his role and put a case together for it. Ian, well aware that he was fortunate to have so much positive support from his hardpressed manager, felt determined to put forward a strong case for developing a service for those with learning disabilities and those who cared for them.

Ian enjoyed the challenge of putting his project together. He developed a creative and forward-thinking proposal that particularly emphasized the role of service users and their carers in the development and evaluation of services. His proposal was adopted, and half of Ian's time was allocated to its implementation. He undertook this with enthusiasm, and such was his success that when a different service wanted to put a case for a new development Ian was asked to help in its preparation. He agreed to do this and again thoroughly enjoyed it, throwing himself into it even though it represented an increase in workload and mainly had to be done in his own time. The combination of his new-found skill and enthusiasm for service development (he was now frequently asked to help with this throughout the social services department) and his work in his job developed Ian's confidence, and rekindled his energy and job satisfaction. He now feels better prepared to look for promotion, recognizing that this may not necessarily be in occupational therapy. Both learning disability and service development generally are now within his grasp.

We can see in Ian's story and in Harjit's and Jeanette's stories, from the previous chapter, people who are energized by the motives that drive them. For all of them, the identity of 'occupational therapist' is important, but the strength of that identity, and the way it is played out in their careers, varies. A concept which captures this commitment and variation is Schein's (1993, 1996) notion of career 'anchors': the attitudes, values, needs and talents that develop over time and which shape and guide a person's career decisions and directions. Whilst they evolve and develop over time as a consequence of real-world work experiences, people's career anchors eventually become a relatively stable part of their psychological make-up. It may take us a long time to establish and clarify what we are really looking for in our work and, of course, we may not always be able to find work opportunities which we view as ideal. Compromises may have to be made. Generally speaking, however, our career satisfaction will be highest when our work enables us to fulfil the criteria of our key work motivations, that is our career anchors. Use the following description of Schein's eight different career anchors in conjunction with Learning Task 9.1 as a framework for considering Ian's career motivations, and also your own.

- *Technical/functional competence:* For the person with this career anchor, the desire for competence in some technical or functional area is paramount. If this is the career anchor that best describes you, you are someone who derives your sense of identity from the exercise of your skills, and you are most happy when your work challenges you in those areas.
- *Service/dedication to a cause:* The motivation of those with the career anchor of service or dedication to a cause is the wish to pursue work that achieves something that they consider to be of value. Helping and enabling others – practically, emotionally, physically – are, of course, all values to which the occupational therapy profession is dedicated.
- *Autonomy/independence:* If your career anchor is autonomy/independence, you like to define your own work in your own way. You like jobs which allow you flexibility in when, where and how you work. You may pass up opportunities for promotion or advancement in order to retain freedom to carry out your work as you wish.
- *Pure challenge:* If your career anchor is pure challenge, you will enjoy working on seemingly unsolvable problems, overcoming difficult obstacles or winning out over tough opponents. The challenge is an end in itself: if something is easy, it immediately becomes boring.
- *Security/stability:* With the security/stability career anchor, the main wish is for financial and/or employment security. Although you may achieve promotion or advancement, you are more concerned with security of tenure than with rank or with the content of your work.
- *General managerial competence:* Here the prime motivation is to rise to a high enough level within an organization to enable you to integrate the efforts of other people and be responsible for the output of a particular department or organization. It is the general area of management that interests you rather than the specific technical or functional area in which you work.
- *Entrepreneurial creativity:* If your career anchor is entrepreneurial creativity, your driving motivation is to create an organization or enterprise of your own, built on your own abilities and the result of your own efforts and willingness to overcome obstacles.

The financial success of the enterprise is important to you as proof, to you and the world, of your abilities.

- *Lifestyle:* Here the key motivation is to integrate personal needs, family needs and career requirements. If this is your career anchor, you define success in terms broader than just career terms, and may be willing to sacrifice some aspects of your career that threaten to upset the balance between the different areas of your life.

Learning Task 9.1   Career anchors

One of the occupational therapists involved in Wright's (2007) study commented: 'I don't *do* occupational therapy; I *am* an occupational therapist'.

In this statement, she is saying something important about what anchors her to her career. Saying she doesn't 'do' occupational therapy does not mean that she has no concern with the technical/functional areas of her work. Rather, she is hinting at something beyond the exercising of her professional skills, something about what her work means to her and how it is a part of who she is as a person. From this we could hypothesize that, in terms of Schein's typology, her fundamental career anchor is 'dedication to a cause'.

Work and career mean different things to different people, and occupational therapy is a profession with a wide range of different types of opportunity to offer its members. Look back to Ian's career story, and those of Harjit and Jeanette from the previous chapter.

- What career anchors can you identify in their career stories?
- Find instances where their career anchors operate together in harmony, and instances where they conflict. How are conflicts resolved?
- In what ways do their career anchors wax and wane?

Now think about your own career anchors. Which ones do you identify with most readily? In terms of their importance to you at the present time, how would you rank the eight career anchors identified by Schein? Is this ordering different from how it would have been in the past? How do you think this ordering may change during the course of your career?

Throughout this work book, it has been stressed that the self is both constant – we are recognizably the same person from cradle to grave – and ever-changing. The change takes place because of growth and experience and, whilst it is individually scripted, it takes place in a life course framework. Professional identity is an important element in many people's sense of self and it, likewise, changes and develops over time. It is not static; we can feel this in Ian's account of his work life. Skovholt (2001), writing principally about counsellors, makes points generalizable to all professions when he identifies several themes characterizing professional development. Three themes of particular interest are:

- As the professional matures, continuous *professional reflection* becomes the central developmental process.
- *Personal life* is a central component of professional functioning.
- *External support* is more important at the beginning of one's career and at transition points.

These themes invoke the life course concepts that have been addressed throughout this work book. The themes emphasize how professional competence is not achieved once and for all but needs to be continually nurtured and kept current. This does not mean, however, that professional development is necessarily a smooth and gradual progression. Rather, our professional development may mirror the alternating periods of transition and consolidation identified by Levinson (1986). Ian's career narrative illustrates this in that he has experienced times of movement and change, and times of consolidation and reflection. If we are to do our best by those we work with, it is important that we build in the re-evaluation points that an evolving life structure requires and make efforts to maintain our own health, well-being and, thereby, our fitness to practise. Skovholt (2001) uses the term 'sustaining the professional self' to describe this process. We can change our career emphasis, or even our profession, whilst still reflecting on where we are, where we want to be and whether our practice is as good as it can be. Ian's narrative shows how professional development can be promoted by seeking and nurturing relationships with suitable professional colleagues. We can also sustain our professional self through explicitly examining the interplay between our personal and professional lives and, above all, through reflective practice.

165

Reflective practice

Reflection involves the process of 'reviewing one's repertoire of experience and knowledge to invent novel approaches to complex problems' (Creek, 1998, p. 66). 'Reflective practice' means thinking about and reviewing what you are doing, taking into account the whole experience – what happened, how you felt, what you thought – and using the process to change things for the better and so improve future practice. Essentially, it is the route by which continuing professional development is achieved, and the Learning Tasks in this work book have been designed to hone your skills in this area. Whilst some of these Learning Tasks focus on what is happening in your life right now, others ask you to look back on past experiences, and are subject, therefore, to the problems of imperfect and incomplete recall. Developing the habit of keeping a reflective diary helps you to capture experience in the moment whilst it is fresh in your memory and before you have, knowingly or unknowingly, placed a particular interpretation on it. This can be cathartic in itself, and can provide rich material for reflection and professional development. A reflective diary provides a record of critical incidents in your professional life, gives a structure to your ideas and monitors the development of your professional thinking. You may well already be in the habit of maintaining this type of journal. If not, then Learning Task 9.2 provides a protocol for doing so.

Learning Task 9.2   Keeping a reflective diary

In order to learn as much as possible from both your positive and your negative work experiences, try to develop the habit of systematically recording and analysing critical incidents from your professional life. A well-thought-through and carefully completed reflective diary can be a valuable professional resource for many years, and it is worth choosing an attractive and robust notebook separate from the Learning Journal that you have developed in conjunction with this work book, and keeping this for use exclusively as your diary.
   Use the directions below to structure your reflections.

* *Recording your reflection*
   ○ Choose a notebook and begin on the second side of the first page, so that you have both a left-hand and a right-hand page to work on.

- ○ On the left-hand page, record incidents from your professional life on a regular basis.
- ○ Still using only the left-hand page, record any immediate thoughts, feelings and comments about the incident.
- *The reflective process*
  - ○ Reread the diary to give you a sense of what happened and how you felt about the whole experience.
  - ○ Using a highlighter pen, or at least a pen of a different colour, highlight anything – positive or negative – that made an impact on you.
  - ○ On the right-hand page, record your present thoughts.
  - ○ Write about the situation, emphasizing how it might have been different or what could be changed next time.
- *Considering what you have learnt*
  - ○ Sum up your learning from this experience.
  - ○ Consider the impression that key experiences have made on you.
  - ○ Consider ways in which your understanding or your values have been challenged or changed.
  - ○ Contemplate where this new knowledge and insight is taking you. How will it affect your future practice?
- *A note of caution*
  It is important to think about who will be reading your reflective diary and to take this into consideration when deciding what to include. Is the diary just for you? Will you use selected extracts for a course assignment, in supervision, or in any other public forum? Will it be seen in its entirety by others: peers, tutors, fieldwork educators, managers?
- Finally, and very importantly, keep your reflective diary safe so that you can both refer back to it and add more material in the future!

Of course, there are many other ways to reflect in addition to maintaining a reflective diary. Both formal and informal discussions with peers, be they colleagues or otherwise, can be helpful. However, it is to supervision, a formal and structured setting for reflection, that our attention now turns.

Supervision

Clinical supervision comprises 'a formal process of professional support and learning which enables individual practitioners to develop knowledge and competence, assume responsibility for their own practice and enhance consumer protection and safety of care in complex clinical situations' (Department of Health, 1993, p. 15). Clinical supervision is essentially a collaborative process between supervisor and supervisee that can fulfil many specific functions, including to teach, counsel, consult, evaluate and monitor professional/ethical issues and to work with the administrative/ organizational aspects of client work (Carroll, 1996). Clearly, therefore, clinical supervision for both students and qualified occupational therapists can play a vital role in developing and maintaining the professional self (Allan & Ledwith, 1998). It is an activity that can be made much more fruitful by the acknowledgement of life course issues in both work practice and your personal life. For example, is work less salient at your particular life stage than it once was or may be in the future? Are you managing a difficult transition in or out of work? Are your colleagues or your supervisor at a very different life stage from you, and does this need bringing into the open so that it can be used to help rather than hinder?

You should try to ensure that you have regular supervision – once a month is usually realistic – and that it is prioritized by both you and your supervisor. The supervisor and supervisee will need to establish clear guidelines about the purposes and nature of the sessions (van Ooijen, 2000), guidelines that may need to be revised over time. Also, what is suitable for one pairing or context may well need alteration for another. It is also the case that the novice practitioner will need a different emphasis in supervision from that required by a more seasoned practitioner (Skovholt, 2001). We have noted in his career story (pp. 160–2) that although Ian was far from a novice practitioner his relationship with his boss, and the honesty within it, was vital to his professional development. Despite some differences in specific supervision needs, there is a similarity in the process and good practice of supervision that is common across settings and relationships. This process of effective supervision can be represented as a five-stage cyclical process (Page & Wosket, 1994; van Ooijen, 2000), as shown in Figure 9.1.

You may find that the sequence of *contract, focus, space, bridge* and *review* engenders in you a sense of déjà vu. Indeed, we rather hope that it does. Like the reflective diary, it has distinct similarities to Kolb's model of experiential learning, which we commended to you right at the start of this work book (p. 2). It can also be seen as a

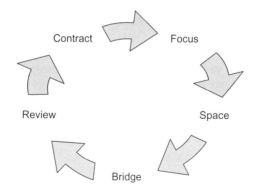

Figure 9.1 Cyclical model of the supervision process (Page & Wosket, 1994; van Ooijen, 2000)

- The *contract* involves the setting of ground rules and boundaries, deciding upon accountability, clarifying expectations and making the supervisor–supervisee relationship explicit.
- The *focus* is important in order to clarify what topics and which aspects of those topics are to be discussed during a session, and priorities need to be agreed, issues and a mode of presentation should be set, objectives decided upon and the approach agreed.
- *Space* is seen as the central part of supervision, and it is within this that issues are explored. There may be challenges and these have to be carefully managed. It is important to recognize that neither clarity nor resolution is guaranteed.
- *Bridge* is where questions are asked which aim to help establish a clearer view and where information may be exchanged; the supervisor's knowledge and experience may be especially useful here. Following this, action can be decided upon and goals set.
- *Review* forms the last part of the session, and within this the session should be evaluated so that sessions can be improved and made more useful. It is helpful to set aside a longer period for review of the whole process every six months or so.

specific use and adaptation of the PMOD framework, which formed the backbone of Chapter 6 (p. 112).

Continuing professional development is a moral imperative for those whose professional work affects the well-being of others. It is also a requirement for registration with the Health Professions Council, the General Social Care Council, the Nursing and Midwifery Council and other professional bodies. We hope that this work book has encouraged and helped you to fulfil this requirement.

The therapeutic use of self

A focus on the life course issues of the health or social care professional rather than (or, more accurately, as well as) the life course issues of the client blurs some of the distinctions between 'helper' and 'helped'. Both are revealed as juggling (perhaps struggling) with issues such as transition, loss, change and role. It encourages recognition of both as similarly human rather than differently placed as 'professional' and 'client'. Such recognition will inevitably be reflected in work with clients, and relates to the therapeutic use of self. The issue of where skills, knowledge and understandings benefit the practitioner and where they benefit the client can become confused: whose interests are really being served when a professional does or does not explicitly call on their own personal experience and self as a basis for understanding and relating with clients? This, along with the associated issue of the appropriate levels of involvement between a practitioner and a client within a successful therapeutic relationship, has exercised the minds of those involved for many years.

In a survey carried out in 1991, using a sample of staff nurses who regularly dealt with terminally ill patients, it was widely agreed that, in terms of becoming therapeutically involved with a patient, reciprocity (that is person-to-person rather than simply professional-to-patient contact) was important (May, 1991). This method of involvement is essentially the employment of the therapeutic use of self. May created a sliding scale of involvement and highlighted the importance of creating a balance whereby therapeutic closeness is tempered by professional distance. He labelled the two end points of this scale *associational involvement* and *demonstrative involvement*:

- *Associational involvement* occurs when the health or social care professional does not offer any level of personal relationship with the patient/client. There is, in effect, no reciprocity. There is an emphasis on technical skills rather than on interpersonal relationships. With associational involvement, the health or social care professional (a nurse in May's case) retains a high level of professional detachment, as was traditionally demanded. Whilst this may protect professionals from becoming emotionally attached to their patients, in maintaining a large professional distance or detachment there is a risk that patients lose any sense of power or influence in relation to managing their condition. They may become alienated from their own treatment, seeing it as out of their control and the responsibility only of their professional carers.

- *Demonstrative involvement*, the other end of the scale, occurs when the health or social care practitioner becomes overly involved with a patient or client. In this instance, empathy and identification with the patient/client mean that the nurse becomes unduly affected by the patient's treatment. Professional distance is lost and the nurse becomes open to hugely increased levels of role stress. Similarly, the patient/client may develop unrealistic expectations about what the nurse, or other professional carer, will or can offer. Demonstrative involvement on the part of the professional carer leaves the patient/client open to almost inevitable disappointment.

Whilst the temptations of associational and demonstrative involvement can be understood – the former offering protection from emotional pain, and the latter the possibility of meaningful personal contact – it is not hard to see that both represent inappropriate extremes. May describes a midway point (incidentally, another 'both-and' position), termed *primary involvement*, that strives both to exploit the advantages of each extreme and to avoid their pitfalls:

- *Primary involvement* occurs when nurses, or other health or social care professionals, find a balance whereby they interact on a personal level with patients/clients but only in order to facilitate the achievement of professional goals. When this is achieved, then the nurse or, indeed, the occupational therapist, will become accustomed to an individual patient's idiosyncrasies and will provide more effective care. Another way of defining primary involvement is as the therapeutic use of self.

As May's scale suggests, an important reason to use oneself therapeutically is in order to create a relationship in which the patient feels that there is trust and authenticity. The importance of this in effective, client-centred working is so great that de Raeve (2002) defines it as a moral necessity within a health professional–client relationship. The patient must feel able to trust and 'know' the professional in order to feel that the relationship, and, indeed, the therapy, is sincere. The therapeutic alliance that is formed between the practitioner and the client has been described as 'the partnership between the therapist and client in which both contribute actively, with mutual respect' (Hagedorn, 2000, p. 311). As such, it is a key to successful intervention.

Whilst the notion of primary involvement can be seen as an effective way of managing the personal–professional boundary between health or social care practitioners and their clients, it has also been suggested that if a relationship requires a health professional to modify or contain their emotions the relationship is inauthentic and untrustworthy. This perspective marks a sharp contrast to the early views of health professional–client relationships as expressed by such researchers as Phillips (1983) and Girard (1988). Phillips, for example, denies that personal friendship or involvement is at all necessary in professional relationships, maintaining that emotional distance is, in fact, essential. This is, in effect, a plea for associational involvement. Both Phillips and Girard are clear that in order to preserve a professional relationship there must be strict limits to intimacy. This is an important reminder that views about the appropriate therapeutic use of self may vary across both health and social care professions and individuals. This will require some tolerance and openness if it is not to disrupt teams and undermine practice. It may also be something that needs to be addressed through supervision and staff development.

Perhaps the importance of the therapeutic use of self is best described by Purtillo (1990). She claims that if one applies the therapeutic use of self successfully, a constructive dependence is created, in which patients realize that, in order to fulfil their goals, they must to an extent depend on the professional. This realization must be built on mutual respect within the professional–client relationship, whereby, and somewhat paradoxically, this dependence leads to freedom. This is the freedom for professionals to do what they see as appropriate in the knowledge that the patient is committed to achieving shared goals, but also the freedom for patients to voice their concerns and opinions, confident in the knowledge that they are more than just another case.

The therapeutic self

Allan and Barber (2005) take a slightly different approach when they focus not on the therapeutic *use* of self but actually on the therapeutic self. They propose that 'there are boundaries between private and professional spheres and that the therapeutic self in this sense is the relationship between the personal and the professional or public self' (p. 392). As such, they offer the possibility of a compromise between the opposing views of de Raeve (2002) and Phillips (1983).

Employment of Allan and Barber's (2005) therapeutic self can be seen as leading to primary involvement. Feelings such as closeness, empathy and unconditional positive regard are observed. Unconditional positive regard – seeing and treating clients as worthy and capable even when they do not feel or act that way – is at the heart of primary involvement. The exercising of unconditional positive regard indicates the use of the therapeutic rather than the personal self, as the health professional's private emotions may need to be suppressed in order to maintain the unconditional positivity that is essential to the professional–client relationship. This idea provides a middle way between unboundaried involvement and a total lack of personal meeting and offers a professional and therapeutic way to take client-centred practice forward. At the same time Savage (1995), writing again about nurses, suggests that use of the therapeutic self facilitates the development of a caring environment that is therapeutic for patients 'without great personal cost for the nurse' (p. 124). This is as relevant for other health and social care professionals as it is for nurses. Unconditional positive regard is no easy achievement, although we would suggest that it, and with it the therapeutic self, can be facilitated by adopting a life course perspective as a framework for understanding the person of both the self (the health or social care professional) and the client.

Use of the therapeutic self, through becoming involved with the person of the client, leads to the attainment of a level of intimacy with clients, but where the only focus of the relationship is the achievement of the client's well-being. The question remains, however, of how a health professional is to set about using this therapeutic self. Hochschild (1983), somewhat controversially, suggests that professionals use a technique called 'deep acting' in order to shape their emotions and feelings appropriately, that is an emotion is shaped to produce a genuine feeling by exhorting a feeling or indirectly using a trained imagination. This deep acting achieves an emotional resonance with the patient which is real for the patient/client but stops short of genuine emotional commitment by the professional. It provides, Hochschild suggests, sufficient emotional linkage and empathy to give an insight into how the client is feeling and responding. Not surprisingly, the notion of deep acting has been both criticized and challenged. De Raeve (2002), in particular, baulks at the notion on moral grounds, claiming that it calls into question the sincerity and authenticity of emotions at the heart of a morally viable nurse–patient relationship.

A middle way has again been proposed by Allan and Barber (2005). They agree with neither Hochschild (1983) nor de Raeve (2002), believing, instead, that emotional closeness or distance depends on natural defences within the health professional that can be put in place in order to avoid their own personal anxieties regarding the patient's condition. Allan and Barber look very specifically at relationships between nurses and fertility patients, in which there are strong emotions at the fore of the treatment. The emotions common in patients at a fertility clinic, those of disappointment and loss, are not dissimilar to terminally ill patients. However, every client is experiencing some degree of trauma and so the findings may be seen to be applicable to most clinical situations. Thus, Sumison (1999) discusses how, in work with older people, the use of the therapeutic self is important in creating an environment of trust. A professional must be intimate at a certain level with a client in order to develop a level of trust that is sufficient for the client to feel at ease in reporting symptoms and circumstances that are potentially embarrassing, and which may range across such varied concerns as incontinence and elder abuse.

Developing and using the therapeutic self is a long-term task and commitment for any health and social care professional. It is something that is likely to figure significantly in your continuing professional development activities. It returns the therapeutic relationship to its rightful place at the heart of client-centred practice and, thereby, the client to their rightful place at the centre of your concern. It is appropriate, therefore, that our final Learning Task – Learning Task 9.3 – asks you to reflect on the therapeutic relationship, including the aspects of your self that you can call on in order to make that relationship therapeutic.

Despite the significance of the therapeutic self and the significance of its use in the client–therapist relationship, it is not the only factor contributing to therapeutic success. It is important to be neither too complacent about relationships with clients that go well nor too self-blaming or critical of relationships that are less satisfactory. Few relationships are a total success or a total failure.

Learning Task 9.3   Effective therapeutic relationships

It is inevitable that you will experience greater levels of success and satisfaction with some clients than with others. This Learning Task invites you to reflect on why this may be so.

- Think about some of the clients you have worked with, either on placement or in your practice. Try to generate a list of five to 10 cases, including instances where you felt your intervention had been successful and satisfying, and instances which left you somewhat disappointed and dissatisfied.
- Taking each case in turn, summarize what were for you the positive and negative aspects.
- Were there elements in the nature of the case that had an impact on how successful and satisfying you felt your intervention to be? Relevant factors may include:
  ○ the nature of the client's condition
  ○ the severity of the client's condition
  ○ the prognosis
  ○ the eventual outcome
  ○ the novelty versus the routine nature of the case
  ○ your degree of involvement: how central you were to the client's treatment and how long you were involved in it
- Describe the relationship that you developed with each of the clients. What were the positive and rewarding aspects for you? What were the more negative or unsatisfactory elements? How do you explain these assessments?
- Where would you place your relationship with each client on May's scale?

1_____2_____3_____4_____5

Associational	Primary	Demonstrative
involvement	involvement	involvement

To what extent and in what ways did the type of involvement you had with the client affect your assessment of the success and satisfactoriness of the case?

Look through your notes and see whether you can identify any themes that characterize those cases you feel most positive about, and those towards which you feel more ambivalent or negative. If possible, compare notes with a colleague who has also completed this Learning Task.

Think about what you have learnt from this activity. Are there any issues that you need to think through further, possibly in supervision?

Relationships may be less than ideal, and yet still achieve something, just as they can be intrinsically rewarding and satisfying and yet fail to achieve all their goals.

It seems self-evident that knowing oneself will help in the planning of appropriate continuing professional development activities that are designed to fill gaps in your knowledge and experience and move you forward. We hope that the issues addressed in this work book will assist you in this task. Such issues include your place on the life course journey in a variety of areas, the current complexion of your life-career rainbow and what is currently most salient in your life, your strengths and weaknesses, your stability zones, your strategies for managing stress and the goals you are trying to achieve. We believe you can use your knowledge of life course theory and life course issues to gain insight into your own practice. Your knowledge and the skills that you have to apply it, both to your work and to other areas of life, can have a significant impact irrespective of your life stage and preoccupations. We hope you have gained something from this work book and we wish you well on your journey.

Key Terms and Concepts

This glossary defines or summarizes the most important terms and concepts used in this book. It also includes a number of terms and expressions whose understanding is assumed or implied, and concepts that you may encounter in your wider reading about the life course and lifespan development. Several of the items could be defined in similar although subtly different ways (see, for example, the glossaries in Bee & Boyd, 2003; Hayslip *et al.*, 2007; Hutchinson, 2008; and Lefrancois, 1999). The definitions given here are those deemed most appropriate for the context in which they are used in the present book.

4-S model of coping effectiveness   Goodman et al's (2006) model identifying four categories of factors influencing a person's capacity to cope with change: the *situation*, *self*, *support* and *strategies*.

Accommodation   The process by which individuals change some aspect of their identity in response to new experiences.

Activity theory   A theory of ageing based on the belief that life satisfaction in later adulthood is promoted by remaining as socially, physically and intellectually active as possible. (See **Disengagement theory**.)

Adolescence   The stage of development between childhood and adulthood that begins with the onset of puberty and typically includes the teenage years.

Ageism   The systematic stereotyping of and discrimination against people because of their age.

Age norms   Sets of expectations, frequently culturally and historically specific, for the behaviour of individuals of a particular age group.

Age structuring The standardizing of the ages at which social transitions occur, by developing policies and laws that regulate the timing of these transitions.

Anonymity Undisclosed identity. This term is usually used in research or in case study work where data are anonymized to protect a person's identity being exposed.

Anticipatory grief The grief reactions experienced before a loss occurs, particularly during the time between learning that a loved one is terminally ill and the actual death.

Assimilation The process by which individuals incorporate new experiences into their existing identity.

Attachment An intimate and powerful emotional bond between two people, notably infant and primary caregiver and from which the child derives security.

Bereavement The process of responding to and coming to terms with the loss of a significant relationship, especially through death.

Biological age The level of a person's biological development and physical health, as measured by the functioning of the various organ systems.

Burnout A state characterized by the feeling that one no longer has the resources to be able to cope (emotional exhaustion), the emotional distancing of oneself from clients (depersonalization) and the feeling that one has achieved little of value (lack of personal accomplishment) (Maslach & Jackson, 1981).

Career anchors The attitudes, values, needs and talents that develop over time and which shape and guide a person's career decisions and direction.

Clinical supervision A formal process of professional support and learning which enables practitioners to develop knowledge and competence, assume responsibility for their own practice and enhance client protection and safety of care.

Code of conduct The code or rules which a member of a profession or other group must adhere to if they are to remain in the profession or group. Such codes are written and overt, and concern ethical and professional behaviour.

Cognition Processes of knowing, understanding, problem-solving and related intellectual activities.

Cognitive development The development of mental or intellectual processes, such as thinking, knowing and remembering.

Cognitive strategies Intellectual procedures used to identify problems, select approaches to their solution, monitor progress and modify responses accordingly.

Cohort A group of individuals born within the same specific period who therefore share the same historical experiences at the same point in their lives.

Cohort effects The effects of social change on a specific cohort.

Concept A single idea based on general notions or a broad abstract principle or way of understanding something

Conceptualization An intellectual process through which concepts (ideas or meanings) are formed.

Confidentiality Not disclosing a person's identity or circumstances. Patients and clients have a right to confidentiality such that their identity and circumstances are known only by a small identified group, or sometimes by only one individual. This term is also used in research or in case study work where data are presented in such a way as to protect a person's identity or circumstances from being exposed.

Congenital Present at birth although not necessarily inherited. Thus, a birth defect would be *congenital* if it were due to the influence of drugs, and *genetic* if it were determined by genetic make-up.

Contextual model A developmental model that emphasizes the importance of environmental variables such as family, school, cohort, culture and historical events. It argues that, in order to explain and understand human development, the context in which development occurs must be considered.

Continuing professional development A continuous process of personal growth focused on improving the capacity and fulfilling the potential of professional people at work.

Continuity People's consistent and continuous sense of who they are over time (*internal continuity*) and/or a continuity of context regarding location, people and activities etc. (*external continuity*).

Convoy A personal network of friends and family members who accompany and support a person through their life course.

Coping The process of managing internal and/or external demands that strain or exceed a person's perceived resources.

Coping strategies Specific cognitive and behavioural efforts to avoid being harmed by particular demands, stresses or strains.

Creativity   The capacity of an individual to produce novel ideas, answers or products.

Crisis   (See **Life crisis**.)

Culture   Learnt behaviour which is socially constructed and transmitted, including family and local norms, peer groups and cohort effects, spiritual, religious, moral and political beliefs, and issues of race and nation.

Daily hassles   Individually relatively small, everyday sources of stress (e.g. mislaying car keys, getting stuck in traffic, running out of mobile phone credit).

Daily uplifts   Individually relatively small, everyday sources of pleasure (e.g. meeting a friend, receiving a compliment, finding mislaid items).

Decision-making styles   Different approaches to decision-making (e.g. *planful, intuitive, compliant*) and the manner in which they are made (e.g. *hesitant, confident*).

Demographic characteristics   Where we 'sit' within our society as a consequence of factors such as our age and life stage, socio-economic status, gender, ethnicity and state of health.

Development   Change across time that involves some systematic improvement, growth, maturation or increase in adaptive capacity.

Developmental tasks   Skills, competencies, activities, milestones etc. that individuals are expected by their culture to accomplish during specific stages of the life course.

Developmental timetable   The average age at which children normally attain a range of observable developmental achievements and which may be used to assess the relative development of individual children.

Disengagement theory   A theory of ageing which holds that it is normal and useful for older people to socially and psychologically withdraw (or disengage) from society, and for society to disengage from the individual. (See **Activity theory**.)

Dual-career family   A family in which both parents develop separate, equally important careers.

Early adulthood   A developmental period that extends from the individual's early or mid-twenties to approximately the mid-forties.

Ecological niche   Bronfenbrenner's (1994) terms for the position of the individual at the centre of a nest of environmental influences that range from very immediate (e.g. family and school) to distant (e.g. general cultural values). It proposes that to understand human development we must understand the interactions that occur between individuals and their contexts.

Elder abuse   Psychological, physical or financial neglect or active harm of older people by others.

Emerging adulthood   A stage in lifespan development (approximately between the ages of 18 and 25 years) that recognizes the multifaceted, provisional, protracted and incremental nature of the transition from adolescence to adulthood.

Empty nest   The stage of parenting when all children have left the family home.

Ethnicity   The sense of belonging to a particular ethnic group.

Experiential learning   Kolb's (1984; Kolb *et al.*, 2001) term for a cyclical process of learning beginning with a concrete emotional experience that forms the basis for reflective observation. Hypotheses are developed from these observations and are actively tested out, a process which, in turn, gives rise to a new concrete experience.

Extended family   A social network of close relatives beyond the nuclear family, for example grandparents, uncles, aunts and cousins. (See **Kinship network** and **Nuclear family**.)

Family life cycle   A sociological term used to describe the steps or stages through which families typically progress (for example marriage, birth of a first child, raising children, raising adolescents, children's departure and dissolution).

Fitness to practise   The competencies and qualities achieved through the successful completion of a programme of training, study or personal development that results in the person who undertakes the programme being fit to practise whatever it is that the programme has offered. All occupational therapy courses where successful students are able to apply for registration with the Health Professions Council need to demonstrate that they lead to fitness to practise in their graduating students.

Flexibility   A flexible style of responding to stress that involves adapting to and complying with external demands and conflicts. (See **Rigidity**.)

Force-field analysis   An approach to managing problem situations that identifies, analyses and seeks to modify forces facilitating change and, in particular, forces inhibiting change.

Gender   Culturally influenced thoughts, feelings and behaviours associated with being male or female.

Gender roles   Culturally defined behaviour patterns associated with and considered appropriate for males and females in a given culture and cohort.

General adaptation syndrome   A sequence of physiological responses to stressors (*alarm, resistance* and *exhaustion*) proposed by Selye (1978).

Genogram   A pictorial display of family relationships.

Grief   An emotional reaction to the loss of a significant attachment relationship such as with a partner, parent or child.

Hardiness   A personality trait that has the potential to buffer a person against stress, and is characterized by *commitment* (the belief that one's life and activities have value and importance), *control* (the belief that one can control events) and *challenge* (the belief that change in one's life is expected and can be beneficial).

Human agency   The use of personal power to achieve one's goals.

Identity   A term often used synonymously with the term *self* to refer to the individual's self-definition (the personal sense of who and what one is). It includes the goals, values and beliefs to which the individual is committed. One of the important tasks of adolescence is to select and develop a strong sense of identity. (See **Self**.)

Infancy   A period of development beginning a few weeks after birth and lasting until approximately the age of two years.

Intentional change   Prochaska *et al.*'s (1992) cycle of intentional change model involves first deciding to make and then implementing behavioural changes: *precontemplation, contemplation, preparation, action* and *maintenance*.

Kinship network   An alternative term for the extended family. (See **Extended family**.)

Late adulthood   The final developmental period, beginning at around ages 65–70 and frequently subdivided into *Early late adulthood* and *Late late adulthood*.

Life-career rainbow   Super's (1980) phrase for a graphic representation of the longitudinal nature of the many roles that individuals may play in the course of their lives. Each band of the rainbow's arc represents a different role.

Life course   The rhythmic and fluctuating pattern of human life over time, marked out by expected and unexpected life events and interactions between the self and the environment. It comprises the unique set of experiences occurring during a person's lifetime.

Life course perspective   An approach to human behaviour that recognizes the influence of age but also acknowledges the influence of historical time and culture.

Life crisis   An identifiable, discrete change, life event or transition whose demands threaten to overwhelm a person's coping resources and often require major readjustments.

Life expectancy   The average number of years a person of a given age can expect to live.

Life review   The internal process by which an individual remembers, analyses and evaluates past experiences in an effort to come to terms with and make sense of personal life experiences. Whilst the life review is generally associated with late adulthood, it can occur throughout life.

Life space   (See **Personal life space**.)

Life space mapping   The process of constructing a mind map of the personal life space. (See **Mind map** and **Personal life space**.)

Lifespan   The theoretical maximum length of an individual life that is unlikely to be exceeded, even with advances in health care and in the absence of accident and disease.

Lifespan developmental psychology   The area of psychology concerned with the description, explanation and optimization of individual development from conception to death.

Lifespan perspective   A view of development that considers it to be a multifaceted, multidirectional, modifiable and lifelong process involving both gains and losses and one influenced by biological, personal, social, cultural and historical influences.

Life structure   A pivotal concept in Levinson's (1986) theory: the overall pattern of a person's life at a given time, including roles, relationships and behaviour patterns.

Life structure evolution   Levinson's (1986) representation of the life course as a sequence of alternating phases of life structure changing and life structure consolidation.

Locus of control   A person's consistent tendency to attribute behavioural outcomes to either internal or external factors.

Maturation   The sequential unfolding of development processes governed by genetic or other biological processes that are relatively independent of the environment.

Mechanistic model   A model of human development based on the assumption that the developmental imperative lies within the environment rather than the person, and that it is useful to view human beings in terms of their reactive, machinelike characteristics.

Menopause   The cessation of menstruation resulting from the physical and hormonal changes associated with the loss of reproductive capacity, and generally occurring during a woman's late forties or early fifties.

Mentor   An influential role model who also serves directly as an informal guide or adviser in relation to the protégé's occupational and/or personal values, goals, behaviours etc.

Metaphor   Describing one thing by saying that it is another, for example that 'life is a bowl of cherries' or that 'the life course is a journey'.

Middle adulthood   The midlife developmental period spanning approximately the ages from 40–45 to 65–70 years.

Middle childhood   An stage in the sequence of development covering roughly the years between the ages of six and 12, that is most of the years of primary school.

Midlife crisis   A personal sense of emotional turmoil that sometimes occurs in middle age as the person re-examines and evaluates accomplishments, goals, priorities and opportunities.

Mind map   A diagram used to represent thoughts, ideas, activities etc. arranged around and linked to a central key word or idea.

Model   A representation of some phenomenon or system, for example the life course or transition process.

Mourning   The culturally and socially prescribed mechanisms for expressing grief following bereavement.

Multimodal-transactional model of stress   Palmer and Dryden's (1995) model of stress that distinguishes seven categories (or modalities) of stress symptoms, responses and management strategies: *behaviour, affect, sensation, imagery, cognition, interpersonal* and *drugs/biology*.

Narrative   (See **Personal narrative**.)

Narrative form   The overall optimistic or pessimistic tone of a personal narrative along with its sense of progression, regression or stagnation.

Nature–nurture debate   A long-standing psychological argument over whether nature (i.e. genetics and biology) or nurture (i.e.

environment and experience) is more responsible for determining development. Whilst contemporary arguments continue, it is now generally accepted that both nature and nurture are crucial, and that it is more constructive to focus on the interplay between nature and nurture than to argue as to the relative significance of each.

Non-normative life events Significant events or transitions that occur in a person's life not associated with any particular age, life stage or historical era.

Normal cognitive decline Age-related decrements in cognitive functioning associated with changes in neurological and physiological functioning that are the normal consequences of ageing. (See **Pathological cognitive decline**.)

Normative life events Significant events or transitions in the life of an individual that have a relatively strong correlation with chronological age and/or historical time.

Nuclear family A family consisting of a mother, a father and their offspring.

'Off time' events Life events whose timing deviates from normative expectations for a particular society. (See **Social clock**.)

Old-old An alternative term for late late adulthood, which, although defined by a reduced level of physical activity and functional capacity rather than chronological age, typically begins between the ages of 75 and 85 years of age.

'On time' events Life events whose timing coincides with normative expectations for a particular society. (See **Social clock**.)

Optimism The belief that problems are temporary, solvable and due to external circumstances.

Organismic model A model of human development based on the assumption that the developmental imperative lies within the person rather than the environment, and assumes it is useful to view people as primarily active rather than reactive, as more like biological organisms than machines.

Palliative care Care of the terminally ill, designed primarily to ease their physical and psychological distress, thereby enabling what remains of their life to be maximally rewarding.

Pathological cognitive decline Age-related cognitive decline associated with illness, trauma or disease that is not an inevitable and irreversible consequence of ageing. (See **Normal cognitive decline**.)

Peer group Individuals of approximately the same age and developmental stage who frequently share common attitudes and interests.

Personal life space An individual and the segment of the social, cultural and material environment that is meaningful to them and with which they interact.

Personal narrative The account of experiences that we construct and tell about our own life in order to provide a sense of identity, meaning and coherence. (See **Personal story**.)

Personal story A particular thread within a personal narrative or an account of a particular experience that is ordered across time according to a theme. (See **Personal narrative**.)

Pie chart A circular chart divided into sections, with each section reflecting relative frequencies or magnitudes such that the size of each section is proportional to the quantity it represents.

Plasticity The capacity of life course trajectories to vary, change and be modified.

Post-traumatic growth Positive psychological change experienced as a result of the struggle with highly challenging life circumstances.

Post-traumatic stress disorder Marked physical and psychological responses to highly stressful or threatening events that persist long after the event and cause clinically significant distress or impairment in social, occupational or other important areas of functioning. Possible symptoms include persistent re-experiencing of the event, persistent avoidance of stimuli associated with the event, a numbing of general responsiveness and/or persistent symptoms of increased arousal that were not present before the trauma.

Problem management and opportunity development (PMOD) A term used to describe a model of effective coping with change that is based on the work of Egan and Cowan (1979) and others that identifies a process of four stages, each with two substages, or steps: *situational review* (*exploration* and *focusing*), *defining preferred scenarios* (*re-framing* and *establishing goals*), *developing an action plan* (*option census* and *programme choice*) and *action* (*implementation* and *evaluation*).

Psychological age The capacities that people have and the skills they use to adapt to changing biological and environmental demands, including skills in memory, learning, intelligence, motivation and emotions. It is also how old people feel.

Psychosocial   Pertaining to events or behaviours that involve both individual and social factors.

Psychosocial crises   Erikson's (1994) sequence of individual/social preoccupations that characterize different stages of the life course and which potentially lead to the development of a significant new personal strength.

Psychosocial transitions   The process involved when an event or non-event results in a change in assumptions about oneself and the world, and thus requires a corresponding change in behaviour and/or relationships.

Reflective practice   The critical analysis and evaluation of one or more work experiences, and the generalization from that thinking in order to improve competence and promote professional development.

Reminiscence   The process of looking back on one's life that occurs at all ages and is a crucial part of the life review. (See **Life review**.)

Rigidity   A style of responding to stress that involves dependence on familiar and well-tried coping strategies, irrespective of whether these are suited to the specific situation. (See **Flexibility**.)

Rites of passage   Ceremonies, rituals and rites that accompany transition from one life stage to another within a culture.

Roles   Sets of expected behaviours and attitudes associated with particular social positions, for example mother, student or occupational therapist.

Role model   A pattern of behaviours that provides an example that can be copied by someone else.

Role-reversal   The reversal of traditional roles, for example when children are called upon to care for their ageing parents.

Self   The sense people have of who they are.

Self-concept   The structured concept that people have of themselves based on their own experiences, the views of others and cultural categories such as race and gender.

Self-esteem   A global sense of self-worth; the belief that one is a valuable, competent, worthwhile person who is valued and appreciated.

Senescence   A degenerative phase of late adulthood marked by physical and cognitive decline and by increased vulnerability to disease and mortality. It begins at different ages for different individuals and is not necessarily characterized by very dramatic changes.

Sensitive period A period of months or years during which specific experiences have their most pronounced effects, for example the first six months of life is a sensitive period for an infant's formation of strong attachment bonds to primary caregivers.

SMART goals Goals characterized by being *specific, measurable, adequate, realistic* and *time-bounded*.

Social age Age measured in terms of age-graded roles and behaviours expected by society; the socially constructed meanings of various ages.

Social clock A shared sense of when certain life transitions, such as completing education, getting married or retirement, should occur and by which members of a society are frequently motivated, or feel pressurized, to comply with.

Socialization The complex process of learning those behaviours and roles that define a given culture. Primary agents of socialization are home, school and peers.

Social support Help rendered by others that benefits an individual.

Stability zone Relatively stable factors in our life that help to anchor us and hold us steady, thereby making it easier for us to cope with large amounts of change, complexity and confusion in other areas.

Stage An identifiable phase in the development of human beings that is often, although not necessarily, age-related.

Stage model of dying Kubler-Ross's (1997) sequence of stages a dying person tends to pass through in coping with their impending death: *denial, anger, bargaining, depression* and *acceptance*.

Stage model of grief Bowlby's (1980) sequence of stages a person tends to pass through in response to loss through bereavement: *shock, pining, disorganization and despair,* and *readjustment*.

Stereotype Frequently unexamined beliefs, attitudes and expectations about individuals based solely on their membership of a particular group.

Story (See **Personal story**.)

Story style The way a personal story is told in terms of it completeness, fluidity and relation to other personal stories.

Stress The arousal of the mind and body when the perceived or actual demands of a situation exceed the individual's perceived or actual capacity to meet those demands.

Successful ageing The maintenance of psychological adjustment and well-being throughout the life course.

Supervision (See **Clinical supervision**.)

Theory An explanation of observations that indicates which facts are important for understanding and which relationships among those facts are most important.

Thought showering A technique for generating multiple and creative options in relation to an issue, idea or problem.

Trajectory A long-term pattern of stability and change based on unique person–environment interactions over time, usually involving multiple transitions.

Transition cycle A relatively predictable sequence of stages a person goes through in response to a significant life event or transition: *shock, reaction and minimization, self-doubt, accepting reality and letting go, testing, search for meaning*, and *integration*.

Transitions (See **Psychosocial transitions**.)

Turning points Events or transitions that result in a fundamental shift in the meaning, purpose or direction of a person's life.

Unconditional positive regard The capacity to see and treat another person as worthy and capable even when he or she does not feel or act that way.

Unfinished business Important things that have been left undone or important feelings that have been left unsaid, often leading to a sense of guilt or regret.

Young-old An alternative term for early late adulthood, roughly between ages 60 and 75, which is often marked by high activity levels and a productive use of time.

References

Allan, F.A. & Ledwith, F. (1998) Levels of stress and perceived need for supervision in senior occupational therapy staff. *British Journal of Occupational Therapy*, **61** (8), 346–350.

Allan, H. & Barber, D. (2005) Emotional boundary work in advanced fertility nursing roles. *Nursing Ethics*, **12** (4), 391–400.

Antonucci, T.C. & Akiyama, H. (1994) Convoys of attachment and social relations in children, adolescents, and adults. In *Social Networks and Social Support in Childhood and Adolescence*, (eds K. Hurrelmann & F. Nestmann). Aldine de Gruyter, Berlin.

Antonucci, T.C. & Akiyama, H. (1995) Convoys of social relations: Family and friendships within a life span context. In *Handbook of Aging and the Family*, (eds R. Blieszner & V.H. Bedford). Greenwood Press, Westport, CT.

Antonucci, T.C. & Depner, C.E. (1982) Social support and informal helping relationships. In *Basic Processes in Helping Relationships*, (ed. T.A. Wills). Academic Press, New York.

Apter, T. (2001) *The Myth of Maturity*. W.W. Norton, London.

Atchley, R. (1999) *Continuity and Adaptation in Aging: Creating Positive Experiences*. Johns Hopkins University Press, Baltimore.

Baltes, P.B. (1987) Theoretical propositions of life span developmental psychology. *Developmental Psychology*, **23** (5), 611–626.

Baltes, P.B., Reese, H. & Lipsitt, L. (1980) Life-span developmental psychology. *Annual Review of Psychology*, **31**, 65–110.

Bassett, H. & Lloyd, C. (2001) Occupational therapy in mental health: managing stress and burnout. *British Journal of Occupational Therapy*, **64** (8), 406–411.

Bee, H. & Boyd, D. (2003) *Lifespan Development*, 3rd edn. Allyn & Bacon, Boston.

Benner, R.N. (1989) *From Novice to Expert: Excellence and Power in Clinical Nursing*. Addison Wesley, Ron Mills, Ontario.

Bichard, Sir Michael (2004) Chapter Three: Children and vulnerable people. In *The Bichard Inquiry Report*. The Stationery Office, London.

Bowlby, J. (1980) *Attachment and Loss Volume 3: Sadness and Depression*. Hogarth Press, London.

References

Boyd, D. & Ellison, N. (2007) Social network sites: Definition, history, and scholarship, *Computer-Mediated Communication*, **13** (1), Article 11. Retrieved 6 November 2007 from http://jcmc.indiana.edu/vol2013/issue2001/boyd.ellison.html.

Bridges, W. (2004) *Transitions: Making Sense of Life's Changes*, 2nd edn. Da Capo, Cambridge, MA.

Bronfenbrenner, U. (1994) Ecological models of human development. In *International Encyclopedia of education*, (eds T. Husen & T. Postlewaite), 2nd edn. Pergamon/Elsevier, Oxford.

Brown, B., Nolan, P., Crawford, P. & Lewis, A. (1996) Interaction, language and the 'narrative turn' in psychotherapy and psychiatry. *Social Science and Medicine*, **43** (11), 1569–1578.

Brown, J.M., O'Keefe, J., Sanders, S.H. & Baker, B. (1986) Developmental changes in children's cognitions to stressful and painful situations. *Journal of Pediatric Psychology*, **11** (3), 343–357.

Bruner, J. (1990) *Acts of Meaning*. Harvard University Press, Cambridge, MA.

Bruner, J. (1991) The narrative construction of reality. *Critical Inquiry*, **18** (1), 1–21.

Bury, M. (2001) Illness narratives: fact or fiction? *Sociology of Health and Illness*, **23** (3), 263–285.

Buzan, A. (2002) *How to Mind Map*. HarperCollins, London.

Calhoun, L. & Tedeschi, R. (2006) The foundations of posttraumatic growth: An expanded framework. In *Handbook of Posttraumatic Growth: Research and Practice*, (eds L. Calhoun & R. Tedeschi). Routledge, London.

Carnall, C.A. (2007) *Managing Change in Organizations*, 5th edn. Prentice Hall, New York.

Carroll, M. (1996) *Counselling Supervision: Theory, Skills and Practice*. Cassel, London.

Clouston, T. (2004) Narrative methods: talk, listening and representation. *British Journal of Occupational Therapy*, **66** (4), 136–142.

Cochran, L. (1997) *Career Counseling: A Narrative Approach*. Sage, Thousand Oaks, CA.

Cohler, B.J. (1982) Personal narrative and the life course. In *Life-Span Development and Behavior*, (eds P.B. Baltes & O.G. Brim). Academic Press, New York.

Cohler, B.J. & Hostetler, A. (2003) Linking life course and life story. In *Handbook of the Life Course*, (eds J.T. Mortimer & M.J. Shanahan). Kluwer, New York.

Cox, T. (1985) *Stress*. Palgrave Macmillan, Basingstoke.

Cox, T. & Ferguson, E. (1991) Individual differences, stress and coping. In *Personality and Stress: Individual differences in the stress process*, (eds C.L. Cooper & R. Payne). John Wiley & Sons, London.

Creek, J. (ed.) (1998) *Occupational Therapy: New Perspectives*. Whurr, London.

Creek, J. (ed.) (2002) Approaches to Practice. In *Occupational Therapy and Mental Health*. Churchill Livingstone, London.

Crossley, M.L. (2000) *Introducing Narrative Psychology: Self, Trauma and the Construction of Meaning.* Open University Press, Buckingham.

Department of Health (1993) *A vision for the future.* Report of the Chief Nursing Officer. HMSO, London.

Department of Health Government (2004) *Choosing Health: Making Healthy Choices Easier,* Foreword. HMSO, London.

Doyle, C.E. (2003) *Work and Organisational Psychology: An Introduction with Attitude.* Psychology Press, Hove.

Egan, G. (2007) *The Skilled Helper: A Problem-management and Opportunity-development Approach to Helping.* Brooks/Cole, Pacific Grove, CA.

Egan, G.E. & Cowan, M.A. (1979) *People in Systems: A Model for Development in the Human-service Professions and Education.* Brookes/Cole, Monterey, CA.

Elder, G.H. (1996) Human lives in changing societies: life course and developmental insights. In *Developmental Science,* (eds R.B. Cairns, G.H. Elder & E.J. Costello). Cambridge University Press, Cambridge.

Elder, G.H., Johnson, M.K. & Crosnoe, R. (2003) The emergence and development of life course theory. In *Handbook of the Life Course,* (eds J.T. Mortimer & M.J. Shanahan). Kluwer, New York.

Erikson, E.H. (1994) *Identity and the Life Cycle: a Reissue.* W.W. Norton, New York.

Erikson, E.H. (1997) *The Life Cycle Completed. Extended Version with New Chapters on the Ninth Stage by Joan M. Erikson.* W.W. Norton, New York.

Ezzy, D. (2000) Illness narratives: time, hope and HIV. *Social Science and Medicine,* **50** (5), 605–617.

Findlay, L. (2004) *The Practice of Psychosocial Occupational Therapy,* 3rd edn. Nelson Thorne, Cheltenham.

Folkman, S., Lazarus, R.S., Pimley, S. & Novacek, J. (1987) Age difference in stress and coping processes. *Psychology and Aging,* **2** (2), 171–184.

Frank, A.W. (1995) *The Wounded Storyteller.* University of Chicago Press, Chicago.

French, G., Cosgriff, T. & Brown, T. (2007) Learning style preferences of Australian occupational therapy students. *Australian Occupational Therapy Journal,* **54** (1), 58–65.

Frye, N. (1957) *Anatomy of Criticism.* Princeton University Press, Princeton.

Gergen, K.J. & Gergen, M.M. (1988) Narrative and the self as relationship. *Advances in Experimental Social Psychology,* **21** (1), 17–56.

Gergen, M.M. (1988) Narrative structures in social explanation. In *Analysing Everyday Explanation: A Casebook of Methods,* (ed. C. Antaki). Sage, London.

Gigliotti, E. (2002) A confirmation of the factor structure of the Norbeck Social Support Questionnaire. *Nursing Research,* **51** (5), 276–284.

Girard, M. (1988) Technical expertise as an ethical form: towards an ethics of distance. *Journal of Medical Ethics,* **14** (1), 25–30.

Goffman, E. (1959) *The Presentation of Self in Everyday Life*. Doubleday Anchor, New York. (Penguin reprint, 1990.)

Goodman, J., Schlossberg, N. & Anderson, M. (2006) *Counseling Adults in Transition: Linking Practice with Theory*, 3rd edn. Springer, New York.

Greenhalgh, T. & Hurwitz, B, (eds.) (1998) *Narrative Based Medicine: Dialogue and Discourse in Clinical Practice*. BMJ Books, London.

Gustafson, J.P. (1992) *Self-Delight in a Harsh World: the Main Stories of Individual, Marital and Family Psychotherapy*. W.W. Norton, New York.

Hagedorn, R. (2000) *Tools for Practice in Occupational Therapy: A Structured Approach to Core Skills and Processes*. Churchill Livingstone, London.

Hagedorn, R. (2002) *Foundations for Practice in Occupational Therapy*. Churchill Livingstone, London.

Harris, R. (1998) *Introduction to Decision Making*. Retrieved 5 September 2007 from http://www.virtualsalt.com/crebook5.htm.

Hauer, P., Straub, C. & Wolf, S. (2005) Learning styles of allied health students using Kolb's LSI-IIa. *Journal of Allied Health*, **34** (3), 177–182.

Havighurst, R.J. (1972) *Developmental Tasks and Education*. David McKay, New York.

Hayslip, B., Panek, P. & Hicks-Patrick, J. (2007) *Adult Development and Aging*, 4th edn. Krieger, Malibar, FL.

Health and Safety Executive (2007) Work-related stress. Retrieved 7 September 2007 from http://www.hse.gov.uk/stress/.

Henkel, M. (2000) *Academic Identities and Policy Change in Higher Education*. Jessica Kinsley, London.

Herr, E.L. (1997) Super's life-span, life-space approach and its outlook for refinement. *Career Development Quarterly*, **45** (3), 238–246.

Hochschild, A.R. (1983) *The Managed Heart: Commercialisation of Human Feeling*. University of California Press, Berkeley, CA.

Holmes, T.H. & Rahe, R.H. (1967) The social readjustment rating scale. *Journal of Psychosomatic Research*, **11**, 213–218.

Honey, P. & Mumford, A. (2006) *Learning Styles Questionnaire (80-item) – Booklet*. Peter Honey Publications, Maidenhead.

Hopson, B. (1981) Response to the papers by Schlossberg, Brammer and Abrego. *Counselling Psychologist*, **9** (2), 36–39.

Hopson, B. & Adams, J. (1976) Towards an understanding of transition: Defining some boundaries of transition dynamics. In *Transition: Understanding and Managing Personal Change*, (eds J. Adams, J. Hayes & B. Hopson). Martin Robertson, London.

Hopson, B., & Scally, M. (1997). *Transitions: Positive Change in Your Life and Work*. Prentice Hall, Englewood Cliffs, NJ.

Hopson, B. & Scally, M. (1999) *Build Your Own Rainbow: A Workbook for Career and Life Management*, 2nd edn. Management Books 2000, Cirencester.

Howard, G.S. (1991) Culture tales: a narrative approach to thinking, cross-cultural psychology and psychotherapy. *American Psychologist*, **46** (3), 187–197.

Hunter, K.M. (1991) *Doctor's Stories: The Narrative Structure of Medicine.* Princeton University Press, Princeton.

Hutchinson, E.D. (2008) *Dimensions of Human Behavior: the changing life course*, 3rd edn. Sage, Thousand Oaks, CA.

Hyden, L.-C. (1997) Illness and narrative. *Sociology of Health and Illness*, **19** (1), 48–69.

Hyson, M.C. (1983) Going to the doctor: A developmental study of stress and coping. *Journal of Child Psychology and Psychiatry*, **24** (3), 247–259.

Jacobs, M. (1998) *The Presenting Past: The Core of Psychodynamic Counselling and Therapy*, *2nd edn*. Open University Press, Buckingham.

Kahn, R.L. (1979) Aging and social support. In *Aging from Birth to Death: Interdisciplinary Perspectives*, (ed. M. Riley). Westview Press, Boulder, CO.

Kahn, R.L. & Antonucci, T.C. (1980) Convoys over the life course: Attachment, roles and social support. In *Life-span Development and Behavior, Volume 3*, (eds P.B. Baltes & O. Brim). Academic Press, New York.

Kahn, R.L. & Antonucci, T.C. (1981) Convoys of social support: A life course approach. In *Aging: Social Change*, (eds S.B. Kiesler, J.N. Morgan & V.K. Oppenheimer). Academic Press, New York.

Katz, N. & Heimann, N. (1991) Learning style of students and practitioners in five health professions. *Occupational Therapy Journal of Research*, **11**, 239–245.

Klass, D., Silverman, P. & Nickman, S. (eds) (1996) *Continuing Bonds: New Understandings of Grief*. Taylor & Francis, London.

Kolb, A.Y. & Kolb, D.A. (2005) Learning styles and learning spaces: enhancing experiential learning in higher education. *Academy of Management Learning and Education*, **4** (2), 193–212.

Kolb, D. (1984) *Experiential Learning: Experience as the Source of Learning and Development*. Prentice Hall, Englewood Cliffs, NJ.

Kolb, D.A. (1999) *The Kolb Learning Style Inventory*, *Version 3*. Hay Resources Direct, Boston.

Kolb, D.A., Boyatzis, R. & Mainemelis, C. (2001) Experiential Learning theory: Previous research and new directions. In *Perspectives on Cognitive Learning and Thinking Styles*, (eds R. Sternberg & L. Zhang). Lawrence Erlbaum, Mahwah, NJ.

Kraut, R., Patterson, M., Lundmark, V., Kiesler, S., Mukopadhyay, T. & Scherlis, W. (1998) Internet paradox: a social technology that reduces social involvement and well-being. *American Psychologist*, **53** (9), 1017–1031.

Kraut, R., Kiesler, S., Boneva, B., Cummings, J., Helgeson, V. & Crawford, A. (2002) Internet paradox revisited. *Journal of Social Issues*, **58** (1), 49–74.

Kubler-Ross, E. (1997) *On Death and Dying: What the Dying Have to Teach Doctors, Clergy, Nurses and Their Own Families*. Simon & Schuster, New York.

Kurtz, L.F. (1997) *Self-Help and Support Groups*. Sage, London.

References

Langford, C.P., Bowsher, J., Maloney, J.P. & Lillis, P.P. (1997) Social support: a conceptual analysis. *Journal of Advanced Nursing*, **25** (1), 95–100.

Lazarus, A.A. (1986) Multimodal therapy. In *Handbook of Eclectic Psychotherapy*, (ed. J. Norcross). Brunner/Mazel, New York.

Lazarus, A.A. (1989) *The Practice of Multimodal Therapy*. Johns Hopkins University Press, Baltimore.

Lazarus, R.S. (1999) *Stress and Emotion: A New Synthesis*. Free Association, London.

Lazarus, R.S. & Folkman, S. (1984) *Stress, Appraisal and Coping*. Springer, New York.

Lefrancois, G.R. (1999) *The Lifespan*, 5th edn. Wadsworth, Belmont, CA.

Levinson, D.J. (1986) A conception of adult development. *American Psychologist*, **42** (1), 3–13.

Levinson, D.J. (1990) A theory of life structure development in adulthood. In *Higher Stages of Human Development: Perspectives on Adult Growth*, (eds C.N. Alexander & E.J. Langer). Oxford University Press, New York.

Levinson, D.J. (1996) *The Seasons of a Woman's Life*. Random House, New York.

Levinson, D.J., Darrow, D.N., Klein, E.B., Levinson, M.H. & McKee, B. (1978) *The Seasons of a Man's Life*. Alfred A. Knopf, New York.

Linares, A.Z. (1999) Learning styles of students and faculty in selected health care professions. *Journal of Nursing Education*, **38** (9), 407–414.

Lynch, G. (1997) The role of community and narrative in the work of the therapist: a post-modern theory of the therapist's engagement in the therapeutic process. *Counselling Psychology Quarterly*, **10** (4), 353–363.

McAdams, D.P. (1993) *Stories We Live by: Personal Myths and the Making of the Self*. William Morrow, New York.

McAdams, D.P. (1997) *Stories we Live by: Personal Myths and the Making of the Self*. Guilford Press, New York.

McGoldrick, M., Gerson, R. & Shellenberger, S. (1999) *Genograms: Assessment and Intervention*, 2nd edn. W.W. Norton, New York.

McLeod, J. (1997) *Narrative and Psychotherapy*. Sage, London.

Mallinson, T., Kielhofner, G. & Mattingly, C. (1996) Metaphor and meaning in a clinical interview. *American Journal of Occupational Therapy*, **50** (5), 338–346.

Maslach, C. & Jackson, S. (1981) The measurement of experienced burnout. *Journal of Occupational Behaviour*, **2** (1), 99–113.

Mattingly, C. (1994) The concept of therapeutic 'emplotment'. *Social Science and Medicine*, **38** (6), 811–822.

Mattingly, C. (1998) *Healing Dramas and Clinical Plots: The Narrative Structure of Experience*. Cambridge University Press, New York.

May, C. (1991) Affective neutrality and involvement in nurse–patient relationships: perceptions of appropriate behaviour among nurse in acute medical and surgical wards. *Journal of Advanced Nursing*, **16** (5), 552–558.

References

Mechanic, D. (1999) *Mental Health and Social Policy: The Emergence of Managed Care*. Allyn & Bacon, Needham Heights, MA.

Miller, M.A. & Rahe, R.H. (1997) Life change scaling for the 1990s. *Journal of Psychosomatic Research*, **43** (3), 279–291.

Miller, S.M. & Green, M.L. (1984) Coping with stress and frustration: Origins, nature, and development. In *Origins of Behaviour*, Vol. 5, (eds M. Lewis & C. Saarni). Plenum, New York.

Murray, K. (1986) Literary pathfinding: The work of popular life constructors. In *Narrative Psychology: The Storied Nature of Human Conduct*, (ed. T.R. Sarbin). Praeger, New York.

Norbeck, J., Lindsey, A. & Carrieri, V. (1981) The development of an instrument to measure social support. *Nursing Research*, **30** (4), 264–269.

Norbeck, J., Lindsey, A. & Carrieri, V. (1983) Further development of the Norbeck social support questionnaire: Normative data and validity testing. *Nursing Research*, **32** (1), 4–9.

Norcross, J.C., Santrock, J.W., Campbell, L.F., Smith, T.P., Sommer, R. & Zuckerman, E.L. (2000) *Authoritative Guide to Self-Help Resources in Mental Health*. Guilford Press, New York.

van Ooijen, E. (2000) *Clinical Supervision: A Practical Guide*. Churchill Livingstone, London.

Open University (1992) *Handling Stress: A Pack for Group Work*. Open University Press, Maidenhead.

Osborn, A.F. (1963) *Applied Imagination: Principles and Procedures of Creative Problem Solving*, 3rd revised edn. Charles Shribner's Sons, New York.

Page, S. & Wosket, V. (1994) *Supervising the Counsellor: A Cyclical Model*. Routledge, London.

Painter, J., Akroyd, D., Elliot, S. & Adams, R. (2003) Burnout among occupational therapists. *Occupational Therapy in Health Care*, **17** (1), 63–76.

Palmer, S. & Dryden, W. (1995) *Counselling for Stress Problems*. Sage, London.

Palmer, S. (1996) The multimodal approach: theory, assessment, technique and intervention. In *Stress Management and Counselling*, (eds S. Palmer & W. Dryden). Cassell, London.

Parkes, C.M. (1971) Psycho-social transitions: a field for study. *Social Science and Medicine*, **5** (1), 101–105.

Parkes, C.M. (1993) Bereavement as a psychosocial transition: processes of adaptation to change. In *Handbook of Bereavement: Theory, Research and Intervention*, (eds M.S. Stroebe, W. Stroebe & R. Hansson). Cambridge University Press, Cambridge.

Pearlin, L.I. & Schooler, C. (1978) The structure of coping. *Journal of Health and Social Behavior*, **19** (1), 2–21.

Pearlin, L.I. & Skaff, M.M. (1996) Stress and the life course: a paradigmatic alliance. *The Gerontologist*, **36** (2), 239–47.

Peavy, R.V. (2004) *Sociodynamic Counselling: A Practical Approach to Meaning Making*. Taos Institute, Chagrin Falls, OH.

References

Pedler, M., Burgoyne, M.J. & Boydell, T. (2006) *A Manager's Guide to Self Development*, 5th edn. McGraw-Hill Education, Maidenhead.

Phillips, D.Z. (1982) Can you become a professional friend? *The Gadfly*, **5** (1), 29–43.

Pickin, C. & St Leger, S. (1993) *Assessing Health Need Using the Life Cycle Framework*. Open University Press, Buckingham.

Pilgrim, D. (1997) *Psychotherapy and Society*. Sage, London.

Prochaska, J.O., DiClemente, C.C. & Norcross, J. (1992) In search of how people change: Application to addictive behaviors. *American Psychologist*, **47** (9), 1102–1114.

Purtillo, R. (1990) *Health Professional and Patient Interaction*. Harcourt Brace, Philadelphia.

de Raeve, L. (2002) The modification of emotional responses: a problem for trust in nurse–patient relationships? *Nursing Ethics*, **9** (5), 465–471.

Reese, H.W. & Smyer, M.A. (1983) The dimensionalization of life-events. In *Life-Span Developmental Psychology: Nonnormative Life Events*, (eds E.J. Callahan & K.A. McCluskey). Academic Press, New York.

Reinert, G. (1980) Educational psychology in the context of the human life span. In *Life-Span Development and Behavior, Volume 3*, (eds P.B. Baltes & O.G. Brim). Academic Press, New York.

Rice, F.P. (2000) *Human Development: A Life Span Approach*, 4th edn. Prentice Hall, Englewood Cliffs, NJ.

Riessman, C.K. (2002) Analysis of personal narratives. In *Interview Research: Context and Method*, (eds J.F. Gubrium & J.A. Holstein). Sage, Thousand Oaks, CA.

Roberts, J. (1994) *Tales and Transformations: Stories in Families and Family Therapy*. W.W. Norton, New York.

Robinson, I. (1990) Personal narratives, social careers and medical courses: analysing life trajectories in autobiographies of people with multiple sclerosis. *Social Science and Medicine*, **30** (11), 1173–1186.

Rodger, B. (2006) Life space mapping: Preliminary results from the development of a new method for investigating counselling outcomes. *Counselling and Psychotherapy Research*, **6** (4), 227–232.

Rotter, J. (1966) Generalized expectancies for internal versus external control of reinforcement. *Psychological Monographs*, 80 (Whole no. 609).

Rotter, J. (1990) Internal versus external control of reinforcement: a case history of a variable. *American Psychologist*, **45** (4), 489–493.

Ruble, D.N. & Seidman, E. (1996) Social transitions: Windows into social psychological processes. In *Social Psychology: A Handbook of Basic Principles*, (eds E.T. Higgins and A.W. Kruglanski). Guildford Press, New York.

Rutter, M. (1989) Pathways from childhood to adult life. *Journal of Child Psychology and Psychiatry*, **30** (1), 23–51.

Rutter, M. (1996) Transitions and turning points in developmental psychopathology: as applied to the age span between childhood and mid-adulthood. *International Journal of Behavioral Development*, **19** (3), 603–626.

Salmon, P. (1985) *Living in Time: A New Look at Personal Development*. Dent, London.

Sandelowski, M. (1991) Telling stories: narrative approaches in qualitative research. *Journal of Nursing Scholarship*, **23** (3), 161–166.

Savage, J. (1995) *Nursing Intimacy*. Scutari Press, London.

Schein, E.H. (1993) *Career Anchors: Discovering Your Real Values*, (revised edn). Jossey-Bass/Pfeiffer, San Francisco.

Schein, E.H. (1996) Career Anchors Revisited: Implications for Career Development in the 21st Century. *Society for Organizational Learning*. Retrieved 15 March 2008 from http://www.sol-ne.org/res/wp/10009.html.

Schlossberg, N.K. (1981) A model for analysing human adaptation to transition. *Counseling Psychologist*, **9** (2), 2–18.

Schon, D.A. (1995) *The Reflective Practitioner*. Arena, Aldershot.

Selye, H. (1978) *The Stress of Life*, (revised edn). McGraw-Hill, New York.

Sennet, R. (2006) *The Culture of the New Capitalism*. Yale University Press, New Haven, CT.

Shanahan, M.J., Hofer, S.M. & Miech, R.A. (2003) Planful competence, the life course, and aging: retrospect and prospect. In *Personal Control in Social and Life Course Contexts*, (eds S.H. Zarit, L.I. Pearlin & K.W. Schaie). Springer, New York.

Shepherd, B. (1999) Possible selves mapping: Life-career exploration with young adolescents. *Canadian Journal of Counselling*, **33** (1), 37–54.

Skovholt, T.M. (2001) *The Resilient Practitioner: Burnout Prevention and Self-Care Strategies for Counselors, Therapists, Teachers and Health Professionals*. Allyn & Bacon, London.

Skovholt, T.M. & Ronnestad, M.H. (1995) *The Evolving Professional Self: Stages and Themes in Therapist and Counselor Development*. John Wiley & Sons, London.

Spence, D.P. (1987) *The Freudian Metaphor: Toward Paradigm Change in Psychoanalysis*. W.W. Norton, New York.

Sugarman, L. (2001) *Life-Span Development: Frameworks, Accounts and Strategies*. Psychology Press, Hove.

Sugarman, L. (2004) *Counselling and the Life Course*. Sage, London.

Sumison, T. (1999) *Client-Centred Practice in Occupational Therapy*. Churchill Livingstone, London.

Super, D.E. (1980) A life-span, life-space approach to career development. *Journal of Vocational Behavior*, **16** (3), 282–298.

Sutherland, V.J. & Cooper, C.L. (1990) *Understanding Stress: A Psychological Perspective for Health Professionals*. Chapman & Hall, London.

Symonds, C.P. (1947) Use and abuse of the term flying stress. In *Air Ministry, Psychological Disorders in Flying Personnel of the Royal Air Force, Investigated During the War, 1939–1945*. HMSO, London.

Tedeschi, R. & Calhoun, L. (1995) *Trauma and Transformation: Growing in the Aftermath of Suffering*. Sage, Thousand Oaks, CA.

Tedeschi, R. & Calhoun, L. (2004) Posttraumatic growth: conceptual foundations and empirical evidence. *Psychological Inquiry*, **15** (1), 1–18.

Thomas, R.M. (1990) *Counseling and Life-Span Development*. Sage, Newbury Park, CA.

Thomas-MacLean, R. (2004) Understanding breast cancer via Frank's narrative types. *Social Science and Medicine*, **58** (9), 1647–1657.

Titiloye, V. & Scott, A.H. (2001) Occupational therapy students' learning styles and application to professional academic training. *Occupational Therapy in Health Care*, **15** (1/2), 145–155.

Tornstam, L. (1989) Gero-transcendence: a meta-theoretical re-formulation of disengagement theory. *Aging*, **1** (1), 55–63.

Tornstam, L. (2005) *Gerotranscendence: A Developmental Theory of Positive Aging*. Springer, New York.

Viney, L. (1993) *Life Stories: Personal Construct Therapy with the Elderly*. John Wiley & Sons, Chichester.

Viney, L.L. & Bousfield, L. (1991) Narrative analysis: a method of psychosocial research for AIDS-affected people. *Social Science and Medicine*, **32** (7), 757–765.

Wenger, E. (1999) *Communities of Practice: Learning, Meaning and Identity*. Cambridge University Press, Cambridge.

Wenger, E. (2003) Communities of practice and social learning systems. In *Knowing in Organizations: A Practice-based Approach*, (eds D. Nicolini, S. Gherardi & D. Yanow). M.E. Sharpe, New York.

Wethington, E., Cooper, H. & Holmes, C.S. (1997) Turning points in midlife. In *Stress and Adversity Over the Life Course: Trajectories and Turning Points*, (eds I.H. Gotlib & B. Wheaton). Cambridge University Press, Cambridge.

Wicks, A. & Whiteford, G. (2003) Value of life stories in occupation-based research. *Australian Occupational Therapy Journal*, **50** (2), 86–91.

Willi, J. (1999) *Ecological Psychotherapy: Developing by Shaping the Personal Niche*. Hogrefe and Huber, Seattle.

Woolfe, R. (2001) The helping process. *The Psychologist*, **14** (7), 347.

Worden, J.W. (1995) *Grief Counselling and Grief Therapy*, 2nd edn. Routledge, London.

Wright, R. (2007) *Professional identity and transition from occupational therapy practice to higher education*. PhD thesis, Sheffield Hallam University.

Index

Page numbers in *italics* refer to tables and boxes; *g* indicates glossary.

client–health professional relationship *see*
  therapeutic self
clinical supervision 167–9, 178*g*
Cochran, L. 132
cognitions 178*g*
  multimodal-transactional model 97,
    99–100, 104, 105
comedy narratives 135–6
competences as career anchors 163
compliant decision-making 109, 110
concrete experience 2, 3, 5–6
concurrent stress and life events 60, 89
conflicting narratives 132
constructive and destructive aspects of
    social networks 67–8
continuing professional development
    160–76, 179*g*
continuity 50–3, 179*g*
controllability of life events 58–9, 63
convoy 47–8, 111, 179*g*
coping effectiveness, 4-S model 56–70,
    101, 177*g*
coping strategies 69–70, 100–5, 179*g*
  change across life course 105–7
creative idea generation *115*, 118
creativity 180*g*
  entrepreneurial, as career anchor
    163–4
  techniques for promoting *114–16*, 118
Creek, J. 166
cultural norms and values as ecological
    niche *33–4*, 35
cyclical models
  of intentional change 63–6, 113,
    124–5
  of supervision process 168–9

decision-making 108–9
  clinical supervision 167–9
  life course context 125–6
  process vs outcome 125
  styles 109–10, 180*g*

see also problem management and
    opportunity development (PMOD)
dedication/service as career anchor 163
deep acting 173–4
demographic characteristics 62, 180*g*
demonstrative involvement 171
Department of Health 167–8
destructive and constructive aspects of
    social networks 67–8
developmental tasks 180*g*
  across life course 22–31, 35–6
  life stage and health issues *27–9*
drugs/biology, multimodal-transactional
    model 97, *100, 104*, 105
duration of life events 60
dying, stage model of 73, *74*, 188*g*

early adulthood *28*, 48, 88, *130*, 180*g*
early childhood *27*, 105–6, 130
ecological niche 32–5, 180–1*g*
Egan, G. 112
Egan, G.E. and Cowan, M.A. 111
emerging adulthood *28*, 88, 181*g*
emotion
  -focused coping strategies 103, 106
  intuitive decision-making 109, 110
  see also affect
entrepreneurial creativity as career
    anchor 163–4
environmental influences in decision-
    making 126
environmental stimuli model of stress
    93–4
Erikson, E.H. 25–6, 62
establishing goals (PMOD) 117
evaluation (PMOD) 122–3
evolving stories 141
experiential learning 181*g*
  and cyclical model of supervision
    process 168–9
  and personal learning styles 2–6
exploration (PMOD) 113

Salmon, P. 144
satirical/ironic narratives 136
satisficing strategies (PMOD) 119
Schein, E.H. 162–4
Schlossberg, N.K. 71
search for meaning 80
security/stability as career anchor 163
self 164–5, 187*g*
  4-S model of coping effectiveness 62–6,
    70, 101
  -concept 50–1, 187*g*
  -doubt 76–7, 137–8
  -esteem/self-worth 22, 30, 187*g*
  -focused coping strategies 102–3, 105
  life events of, and others 55–6
  see also therapeutic self
Selye, H. 94
sensations, multimodal-transactional
    model 97, *99*, *104*, 105
service/dedication as career anchor 163
setting as ecological niche 32–4
shock
  general adaptation syndrome 94
  and immobilization 74–5
situation
  4-S model of coping effectiveness
    57–61
  -focused coping strategies 102–3, 105
  review (PMOD) 112–14, 123
  see also entries beginning environmental
skilled helper model 112
Skovholt, T.M. 152, 157, 165, 168
  and Ronnestad, M.H. 148, 152
SMART goals 117, 188*g*
social clock 131, 188*g*
Social Readjustment Rating Scale 93
social support 22, 44, 46, 188*g*
  4-S model of coping effectiveness 66–9,
    70, 101
stability narratives 135
stability zones 43–6, 188*g*
  loss of 82, 140–1

stability/security as career anchor 163
stage models
  of dying 73, 74, 188*g*
  of grief 73, 74, 188*g*
stories *see* narratives
story style 139–42, 188*g*
stress
  concurrent, and life events 60, 89
  definitions of 92–6, 189*g*
  indicators of *99–100*
  management *see* coping strategies
  models
    environmental stimuli 93–4
    multimodal transactional 97–100,
      103–5, 184*g*
    process 95–6
    response 94–5
  symptoms of 96–7
Super, D. 15–16, 17
supervision, clinical 167–9, 178*g*
support
  and professional functioning 165
  see also social support
Symonds, Sir Charles 94

technical/functional competence as
    career anchor 163
Tedeschi, R. and Calhoun, L./Calhoun,
    L. and Tedeschi, R. 82, 84–5, 86
testing 79–80
therapeutic self 172–6
  use of 170–2
Thomas-MacLean, R. 138–9
time constraints in decision-making 126
time management 103
timing of life events 58, 91, 131–2
tragedy narratives 136
transitions
  dynamics of 73–81
  and turning points 71–3
  see also loss; stress
triggers for life events 58

unconditional positive regard 173, 189*g*
unspoken stories 141

values
  as ecological niche *34*, 35
  as stability zones 44

Wenger, E. 148, 152, 157
Wetherington, E. *et al.* 72
Wicks, A. and Whiteford, G.
  143–4
Woolfe, R. 52–3
Wright, R. 36, 145, 164